BOOK DESCRIPTION

Letting go can be one of the hardest things you will ever do, and so to avoid more pain, you may be holding onto things that no longer serve you. When you let go of things, it doesn't mean your loss is now "okay." Instead, it means you are going to be okay.

Join Julian on this journey of inner peace, wellness, and finding your release from loss as she guides you through the steps of letting go. Sharing her tragic losses and how she managed to find her way to inner freedom, Julian guides you on a path of personal letting go and healing.

No matter the loss you may have suffered, you can benefit from learning how to let go, heal, recover, and move forward instead of moving on. If you have suffered:

- The loss of a parent, child, or spouse
- The pain of breakups
- The devastation of divorce
- The agony of failing on your life's journey

Then *How to Let Go of Someone You Love: Deal, Heal & Forgive After Loss* is for you.

Armed with the action steps of this journey, you can begin to:

- Prepare to let go
- Discover acceptance
- Embrace change
- Stop harmful behaviors
- Unleash the power inside you
- Move past letting go and create a future instead of living in the past

If you or someone you love is in the painful valley of loss, you need the gift of letting go. Develop this precious talent today with *How to Let Go of Someone You Love: Deal, Heal & Forgive After Loss*!

HOW TO LET GO OF SOMEONE YOU LOVE

DEAL HEAL & FORGIVE AFTER LOSS

JULIAN DEMARCO

ISLAND HAMMOCK PUBLISHING, LLC

CONTENTS

As a way of saying thank you for your purchase and giving back, I'm offering a free Wellness E-Book complimentary with this book exclusively for our readers. You will discover a workbook with action items, exercises, and identifiers to assist you on your path to recovery and healing. This workbook is not available in stores or anywhere else online. Everything that you need to heal on your way to taking back control of your emotions starts here. Go to www. juliandemarco.com to download your free Wellness Workbook E-book! Your patronage is sincerely appreciated!

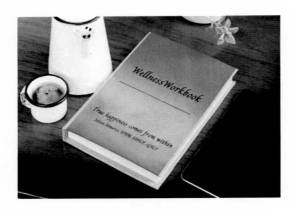

For my three daughters, for having faith in me.
To my momma and Aunt Joyce for the support you've
given that lit the fire within me.
I love you!

INTRODUCTION

Some of us think holding on makes us strong; but sometimes it is letting go.

— HERMANN HESSE

Letting go is one of the most painful and heart-wrenching of experiences. Whether someone has passed from this life or whether they have "only" left yours, letting go is an act of courage that far exceeds that of hanging onto them.

I've certainly had my share of those "wanting to hang on, but needing to let go" moments, as have we all. It hurts, and it's that deep, ever-present aching pain that doesn't seem capable of ever leaving you. But the question is: can you leave it? Can you free yourself from pain and loss?

Loss ...

Such a sad four-letter word that hardly seems capable of explaining the complicated feelings we have when something or someone we love leaves our lives or this life. As a child, you probably experienced your first sense of loss when you had to face up to a grandparent passing away or a much-loved pet dying. Perhaps you had a friendship end at a tender age, but regardless of the type of loss, the result was the same: deep and aching loneliness. You were left with a void to fill where that person, animal, or friend had been.

Often, instead of moving on, we hang around in a state of limbo, hoping against reality that the presence we have lost from our lives will miraculously return, and everything will be right as rain. It doesn't happen. And soon, we are left with the gloom of an endlessly rainy life, all gray and drab.

For children, this is devastating. Usually, death is something they experience with a beloved pet's passing. The pain is numbed by parents buying another goldfish (after the toilet ceremony) or a new puppy when the old dog has passed. This action establishes a sense of continuity in the young child's life.

When you're an adult, the loss you experience will be more lasting. Who will "buy" you a new lover, child, parent, or friend who has moved or passed away? The loss lingers, and you become stuck in this endless moment of being without them. Somehow, it would be best if you found the strength to let go, to move on, to begin anew, and to continue with your life, despite the devastating changes you have suffered.

Yet, doing just that can be a real challenge when you have become entrenched in the pit of despair. How do you move on, and how do you let go when you have just lost someone you treasured? It may seem like the person who left has taken a part of your soul with them, leaving you forever wounded. Even if it's "only" a break-up, you may feel like you have lost everything that mattered to you, and the road ahead becomes unimaginable. Inertia sets in, and soon, you are utterly trapped and stuck. What now?

It was difficult after the breakup of my fiancé and me, whom I loved so dearly. He was able to get to me more than anyone had before. Not everyone knew the "why" we were no longer together, so taking down our photos was hard to do but necessary. You could see just how happy and in love we were in them, especially photos after he proposed to show my beautiful ring. I was hurting after he was unfaithful, and I needed not to be reminded of what was lost. We had remained friends saying once my trust was restored, we'd get back together.

Time passed, and we did, but it was no different than it was before. I knew that I deserved better and to be happy. The heartbreak was the same, and I need to let go of all maybes and wishful thinking. History had repeated itself, and some people just don't change. Beginning the process again was easier since I'd been here before. It didn't hurt any less, no that was ever prevalent and seething, but I wasn't going to allow that to overshadow the other joys in my life like I had allowed it to previously. I valued myself even if he didn't. There's a saying that sometimes people are just beneath you. So, with that thought, I stood up, dusted myself off with my head held high, and began the process of letting go for the final time.

I'M SORRY

When I first suffered debilitating losses, I was always utterly perplexed and wholly annoyed by other people's expressions of "I'm sorry." It was a nice gesture, sure, although it certainly wasn't helpful. Having suffered through my parents' unexpected divorce as a child and being separated from my mother for a time, I have certainly known the bitter taste of loss.

My first significant loss was my stepfather to cancer, whom I loved very much. He raised and treated me as if I was his biological daughter and was the love of my mother's life. I felt a strong urge to drive up to Michigan for Thanksgiving just weeks after giving birth to our daughter. My husband made no complaint about driving the twelve hours up there in the sleek and the snow. We spent two weeks with momma and dad, and how happy he was to hold his new granddaughter. Our time flew by, and before we left, I told dad how much I loved him and thanked him for being so good to me. Dad died the day after Christmas. My first dealings with parental loss and was a hard pill to swallow.

Those losses were terrible enough, but then I lost my unborn child, and the futility of life seemed to overwhelm me as I suffered induced labor to remove my stillborn son. Holding his perfect tiny body in my hands with his green eyes, blonde hair, ten fingers, and ten toes, I couldn't wrap my brain around the tragedy of losing someone so perfect and completely without reason. There was no why. No reason for his death at all. He was perfect in every possible way, but he didn't live.

I forced myself to carry on. And there was nothing anyone could say that eased my pain or lessened my suffering. I managed to persevere right into my divorce on my birthday and then a phone call that would shatter my world. My stepmother called, not to tell me happy birthday, but that my father had been diagnosed with Lou Gehrig's Disease, ALS (amyotrophic lateral sclerosis). The doctors gave him two years to live. I had no idea what this was, and I certainly didn't expect this news on my birthday.

Terrified, I looked it up, and two words hit me like a sledge-hammer to the heart: incurable; fatal. I was dumbfounded! How in the world did this happen? Why wasn't it diagnosed sooner? The day I decided to divorce my husband, I was told my father had an incurable disease? I felt as if I were in the "Twilight Zone" show where nothing made sense. After more tests the following day, the prognoses worsened, and his time left lessened. The call came in from my stepmother, saying that I needed to come to say goodbye to him and that he was fading fast. Questions ran through my mind about how this is possible. The doctors just diagnosed it two days ago! How is it that he's now at the end?! I rushed to gather my things to make the hour and a half drive to him, hoping to say goodbye and tell him something I had been holding back for a long time. I wanted nothing more than to say these words to him, but I was too late. She called before I could even get out of the door, telling my husband that daddy was gone. I accused him of lying to me just to be mean and keep me from leaving so that we could "talk" more.

His death was the truth, and I missed the chance to say a proper goodbye as I did for my stepfather, but most of all, the words that he had wanted most in the world from me. That I forgave him for not being there for me when I needed him and, in his words, being a bad father. I held this rage inside myself for a very long time, and each year around my birthday, I would sob and slump into a devastating depression.

The loss of both of my fathers, a child, and the break-up of relationships have brought many attempts at placations or consolement from people trying to offer comfort. Most failed terribly in this, causing me more pain instead. Perhaps you may even have faced a few of these:

- I'm sorry for your loss.
- If there's anything I can do, just let me know.
- Oh, it's so sad that things didn't work out between you and so and so, but you're better off without them.
- I kind of saw this coming. They weren't deserving of you.
- I'm so sorry your child passed. You can always have more.
- It's an ending to your parent's suffering to pass on. They're no longer suffering.

While all of these offerings of condolences were well-meaning, none of them helped. Yet, people feel like they need to offer you some advice or somehow show they can understand your loss. But here's the thing: it's *your* loss, just like it was *my* loss. Most of the time, they can only sympathize with you unless they'd experienced the same type of loss. But still, people usually feel the need to ask if there is anything they can do for you. Unless they can mend the hole in your heart, then no, no amount of hot chocolate, ice cream, or shopping spree will help.

In the beginning, when I was dealing with my pain, I would vehemently defend "my" grief, believing I was the only person on earth to have suffered such pain. Yes, it may sound immature, but when you are in unbearable life-stopping pain and suffering loss, you tend to think you are the only one who has endured it. Somehow, it makes you unique, and in feeling special, you permit yourself to wrap yourself up in your pain thoroughly. You become a hermit from the world.

You don't want to hear "I'm sorry," and you don't want to be counseled or guided. You just want to live in this moment of deep and dark pain as that, at least, seems to reflect what you are feeling. Oh, and that pit of deep despair is endless. It's so intensely deep that it tunnels right through your life. Soon, if you don't find your way out, you will become a ghoulish version of yourself.

That is the truth I discovered. I finally took a long and hard look at myself, at my pain and my self-consuming grief. I realized I had to change. I feared that if I allowed myself to let it go, the memory of them would also fade. I knew that I had to let go before there was nothing left of me to share with those still in my life. The dead and those who had chosen to walk away no longer had use for me, but I still had use for me. My children still had use for me, and when my heart was ready to heal, the new people who entered my life would as well. I was still valuable. You are valuable too.

Grief as a Process

I realized that grief, letting go, and moving on was not something you just decided to do. You spend months, even years, building a relationship with the person who had left your life, and expecting that relationship to fade away overnight was not realistic, nor was it helpful. Instead, I began to realize the process of grief. By learning how to let go of someone I loved, I found my mile marker that signaled my return to life and the joy of living. As with grief, there is a process to go through for the loss. It wasn't easy, but taking the first steps is crucial. It doesn't mean that the loved one is gone from your life. It is the pain of losing them. I want to share my insights and hard-earned knowledge with you here in hopes that you will benefit from my experience.

When I was processing my grief and creating my journey to self-recovery, I began to research how other people dealt with their grief, how they let go, and how they had moved on. I started studying psychology and human behavior further, and later in dealing with trauma from childhood, I found NLP (neuro-linguistic programming) that changed my life. With a deep desire to help others overcome trauma after healing myself, I became a certified Practioner in NLP. My quest to find answers led me to a process that guides you through the aspects of letting go:

- The beginnings of letting go
- Beginning with yourself
- Embracing change
- How to stop the downward spiral
- Dealing with what's inside yourself
- Initiating and seeking change
- Beyond letting go
- Forgiveness and the past

I know pain, and I know sorrow. While I won't offer you any soft, soapy words to cheer you up or tell you to get over it and move on, I can provide you with the guidance of my own experience with grief, loss, and life after losing someone you love. Letting go *is* possible, and you can find your way forward to healing, dealing, and forgiving after loss. I won't say I'm sorry—I know it doesn't help. I won't tell you any of the unhelpful offerings you may have heard before. But I will stretch out my hands and my heart to you. Both have seen great pain and grief, but I have taken my destiny in my own hands and healed my heart, and you can do it too. I offer you all of the experience and skills from my education that I have amassed in dealing with grief, and your healing is possible right now

But where to start? We'll start at the beginning taking the life out of the rear-view mirror and head into the future with both eyes on the road ahead.

1

THE BEGINNING

Nothing in the universe can stop you from letting go and starting over.

— GUY FINLEY

When you've suffered loss, you are stuck. It's like a wall suddenly springs up before your eyes, and you simply can't see a way forward. Your world stops while everyone else continues living around you. It may seem so incredibly unfair that the world continues while your life has ground to a halt.

Instinctively, you may know that you have to let go. You know you need to move forward even if you can't move on.

All of this starts with acceptance. It's going to be hard; I won't lie to you. However, it's worth it. I understand that burying it, not dealing with it, is an option, but we all know nothing stays buried for long. We also don't have the option of a fast-forward remote to speed through the process, not to have to endure the pain, but we know that's not realistic either.

The first steps are the hardest because we don't want to feel pain. It's in our nature not to want to do this, but we must do it ourselves. You may feel so distraught that you believe you're too broken to move past this or the other feeling, being numb. I will repeat a phrase several times throughout this book that became my foundation when I felt I couldn't endure anymore and because it's the truth. *"You are stronger than you give yourself credit."* I know you may want to curl up in a ball and just die. It feels as the world has shattered and like you're in pure hell. I know that feeling very well, and I've been where you are more times than I'd like to admit so, I feel for you. I'm here to tell you that you can and will get through this. It takes time, so give yourself some room to breathe. With that said, let's take a deep, cleansing breath and start the journey towards healing so you can let go. You've got this!

THE MEANING OF LETTING GO

What does it mean to let go? We have this idea in our minds that letting go of loss means we wake up one morning, and everything is just A-okay and right in the world, and we can carry on like nothing wrong had happened before. It isn't what letting go is at all.

Letting go of loss means you liberate yourself from the past, and you embrace the present as your new reality and acknowledge this "now" as the time where you live. It's imperative to realize you need to release your painful past before living in the present. You can't step forward when you have a foot planted in the past.

I always like to think of this process of letting go as someone who is trying to catch a fish, but their hands are loaded with the smaller catch they made before. They can only catch the larger fish swimming past them to let go of the small fish still locked in their hands. Likewise, when you want to let go of loss, you need to make sure your hands are free from the past and open to taking hold of your present and your future.

Letting go doesn't mean:

- You write off the person whose love you have lost through death or moving out of your life. Instead, you release the pain of that loss and open yourself up to the love of new people who are coming into your life (or may already be there).

- Your pain is fake or imagined. It's about you letting go of the pain and the beliefs that have made that pain linger. You allow a new, helpful, and hopeful belief system to form, which will guide you to a healthier future.

- You are all better tomorrow. Rather, it means you take steps every day to become better, heal, and slowly permit yourself to move on (even if that moving on is inch by inch).

When you aren't ready to let go, you cling on. It can be devastating to your life and happiness as you begin to believe your negative thinking. You are no longer in pain; instead, you are pain. It's in everything you do and in everything you see. It may be all you think about is this loss and pain. If you don't start the journey of self-healing, you will begin to disintegrate your inner self self-talk with negative emotions, eventually resenting what you lost.

By all means, you should grieve a loss. It's an end to what you knew, how you lived, and at times, had become your identity. But grief isn't infinite. There is no "nobility" in grieving. Instead, you need to allow yourself time to heal, then move forward. Hanging on means your hands are so packed with your own pain that you can't catch the beauty all around you.

Hanging onto your loss and your grieving means you will begin to:

- Attach to negative feelings, becoming that rage, hate, disappointment, or anxiety.
- Think negative thoughts, sometimes even about the person you lost. I recall how (in my deepest & darkest moment) I started to wish that I had died with my stillborn son since that would somehow spare me the agony I was suffering now.

Healing from that loss was an enormous process, and in the end, I could release that pain into the past so I could continue into my future, living for my young daughter.

- Feel shame at the resentment you are starting to create in yourself towards everything and everyone in your life.

I remember feeling such shame because I tried to convince myself that my father had been a lousy parent all of the time. In my grief-muddled mind and, hate to admit it, I began to think that it wasn't so bad that he was gone. It meant I no longer had to forgive him for how he hadn't always been there for me. That shame ate at me big time!

I had to let go of that loss, the negative feelings, and self-talk that dominated me to begin to truly forgive my father, not in the act of desperation, and celebrate his life without reservations.

We have to accept that our reality is no longer the wish that we had. My father would never bounce his grandchildren on his knee again, and I had to admit that truth and move forward. It required that I create a new reality that gave me a life purpose and joy at being alive. In clinging to the past and the pain, I was fighting against my reality.

I realized over time how exhausting this was. Instead of making the most of it, fighting is like closing your hands to blessings instead of opening them. I had to take a hard look at the thoughts that dominated my mind, as these thoughts were keeping me from embracing the now. I had begun to believe that my loss was always wrong. But was this true?

My loss had not always been bad. Painful as this was to process, I realized that even death served a purpose. Yes, my father had been suffering, and his passing was an end to that pain. Was it fair that he developed a terminal illness? No. However, was it helpful to only focus on the tragic loss we experienced with him only living two days past his diagnosis and focusing on his death? Or could I instead recall the years before that and carry that power with me? My focus had made me a victim instead of living a life within my ability to control.

Letting go meant something unique for me. I had to release the feeling of the blame for my own anger at my father's death. His death wasn't my making, and I hadn't been responsible for the death of my son before he had even known life. But what I did hold was the power of moving forward and my responsibility. With this change in thinking came acceptance.

ACCEPTANCE

When you start to realize you need to move forward, you can't linger in your grief endlessly, and you begin to prepare for acceptance. While this is known as one of the stages of grief, I have come to understand the grief stages to be cycles that interact and reoccur as you need them to. You give yourself permission to lift your eyes from your sorrow and look ahead in life with acceptance. That isn't to say your loss is now "okay." It will never be, but you will be okay. Although it may be all-consuming, you will be able to make it through. "You are stronger than you give yourself credit."

There are a few elements of your grief that you need to accept for healing to begin. When you acknowledge the pain, you can separate it from yourself. Grief and loss can make you become a part of your pain, which leads to suffering. You are more than the sum of your pain. Let go and accept that pain has happened, and you now have a choice between being a victim or taking control of your life. I found acceptance had many aspects, which I had to learn. My journey allowed me to start to develop acceptance:

Of Truth

One of the hardest things to accept was that I had moved into a new reality without the person who had moved away or passed. In some instances, you may need to accept the truth that while the person may still be in your life, they are no longer part of it. It can be enormously painful as there is no final resolution to losing someone you loved, but now you are separated.

In my own experience, I had to accept my own traumatic past, a past that started in my early childhood with sexual abuse, cascaded through parental loss, and was followed by divorce and finally domestic violence. These traumatic events shaped me, and I continued to wish they had never happened for the longest time. I had locked myself in place to be a victim forever because I tried to bury them so that they couldn't hurt me any longer. In this form, I attempted to dissociate myself to feel no emotions towards the memory by suppressing it as if it hadn't happened. Unfortunately, not dealing with it kept me in a perpetual state of Association-having feelings attached to memories as if they were fresh and just occurred. They also brought with them anxiety, nightmares, and panic attacks that ran in my subconscious mind. I was on a loop feeling the loss over and over, and in a sense, I had become my abuser by not letting myself accept the truth that I was no longer in those situations. I wasn't in the past, and I could finally accept that the pain and trauma *were* in the past. I could only begin to let go as long as I lived in the truth of the present.

In doing so, it brought me a unique insight into what I had experienced. I began to realize the painful and liberating truth: I wouldn't be who I was today without those experiences (traumatic as they were). They had molded me, but they didn't define who I am at my core. By resenting my past, I was resenting myself. Letting go in this example meant freeing myself from self-blame and positively taking steps forward.

Later on, I learned techniques from NLP (neuro-linguistic programming) that I wrote in another book titled "Understanding Childhood Trauma & How To Let Go." This type of therapy allowed me to acknowledge what happened during my traumas and heal, no longer emotionally tied to them. However, it was complex as pain usually is. My history and experiences made me grow and influenced the shift in my life and my career. So accepting doesn't mean that you just lay down and let it bulldoze over you. It's all about seeing it for what it is and coming to terms with it, learning what you can from it then move forward.

To practice acceptance, you need to develop self-honesty. We are great at spinning half-truths to keep ourselves locked in our victimhood, so being honest is the first step towards truth and moving on. That doesn't mean you trivialize what happened in your past. It simply means you give yourself permission to look at it and realize that the pain or personal loss is no longer here with you. You recognize the one who keeps torturing you with the loss and pain is *you*. However, you have the power to choose to let go, move on, and truth-fully look at who and where you are now.

Of Fear

So, why do we hold ourselves back? Why do we continue to dwell on our loss instead of looking towards our futures as if we're gluttons for punishment? Is it simply easier to live in misery? It's a short answer: our fear causes and perpetuates suffering. That pain is all we know, and we tend to hold onto it like it's the best gift ever. Ironically, the best gift is to let go.

Fear holds you back. It clouds your thinking, and in the words of the *Dune Saga*, "fear is the mind-killer." When fear is your daily companion, you become unable to see ahead, and you can't imagine any type of future, which leads to you being afraid even to try. Fear is that negative self-talk that echos the words said to you that you're not good enough, you can't do it by yourself or that you'll fail; therefore, you fail in self-fulfilling prophecies.

I didn't know how to continue with life after my divorce, despite being an unhappy marriage. It had become all I knew —servitude and not standing on my own two feet for fourteen years. Still, my fear was the real culprit, telling me that the future was worse than what I had suffered in an abusive relationship. In my head played the loop that I was dumb and that I would never survive on my own, along with a string of other falsehoods. Once I managed to handle my fear and the negative self-talk, I realized the future wasn't where fear lived. Fear lived here, right now, and it was tying me down.

Part of that fear was also the fear of being rejected. Someone had died, thereby proving (to my often-emotional mind) they no longer wanted to share their life with me, and even divorce was the ultimate expression of not being good enough. Although the divorce decision was mine, that loss had become a judgment of my worthiness of being a "good wife." With that said, and if you're honest with yourself, you know in your heart that you are also dealing with this same fear deep inside that influences your internal belief system. The loss triggered it, and now you fear losing more and may feel like a failure; you're not.

While fear can be a good thing that makes you slow down and examine life aspects closer, it can also act like a bridge that appears broken that halts you completely. You can't see a way to get over it, and you don't have faith or believe in your ability to get to the other side. What you don't see is that the bridge is indeed intact, and it was your perspective that made it appear uncrossable.

I had to believe in myself, knowing that I held power to nurture the light within, even though it felt that it had gone out. Fear no longer had any control over me once I became brave enough to lift my eyes and look ahead in life. Fear makes you doubt your self-worth and is like a thief in the night that robs you of energy causing you to stagnate in your life.

I began to write extensively about all the things that had me wrapped up in fear. It was a painful but strangely liberating exercise, and after a few weeks of writing about every single worry, anxiety, and "what if" that had so dominated my life, I realized I had the power to move past all of them once I accepted it. You can do it too. My experiences with fear, letting go, and acceptance is something I would love for you to explore in your own life, and I guide you through this process of writing in the first of the action steps in this book.

Of Letting Go

When I had unmasked my fears, I began to accept that I could let go of the things that had weighed me down. I had the right to a life without the weight of my baggage. Oh, I'm not saying you need to toss your baggage by the wayside. You are, after all, shaped by your experiences, but you can choose not to carry a whole trainload of unpleasant souvenirs on your life journey because they don't define you. You can keep a few postcards, and it's up to you to decide what you will save and what you will put into storage or donate to the past. Not everything needs to go with you into the future to your next destination in life.

I accepted that it was okay to let go of things that no longer served a purpose in my life. That was significant for me. Can you imagine finding the things that don't help you in your life and simply thanking them, folding them up, and sending them off on their way? What freedom this brings!

With freedom comes an improved energy flow. After all, when you hang onto things, you block energy in your life, and you will pay the price with fatigue and emotional strain disabling you. When I began to let go of things I no longer needed, I felt energized, and I could start to live my life again, dancing, spending time with my children, and later with my grandchildren. I could once again offer care and love to those who mattered in my life instead of wasting them on people who no longer cared or were beyond the living world.

AWARENESS OF SELF

With acceptance came self-awareness, and I felt interested in my life again. With time and sustained work, I began to enjoy my life. You can move from grieving and loss to forward vision and enriched life. Where everything had hurt, I could now start to carefully analyze what hurt, what was anger, and find where I had hidden my joy.

I had to rediscover my feelings. I guess the only way to describe what this means is to tell you about the time I hit my foot on the edge of my bed. You've probably done it too. Walking in a dark room, and there, smack! Your little toe locates the usually out-of-the-way edge of your bed. The pain is indescribable. It seems to multiply and make your whole body ache until you don't know what is actually hurting. It may be your toe, but it may also be your ear lobes. Everything hurts, and you don't know how the rest of you feels. There is just pain.

This is what a sudden and overwhelming loss *feels* like. It hurts everywhere. When you are in this much pain, you lose track of all the other feelings you have. They kind of muddle together into an aching numbness instead of letting you see your pain, experience your anger and acknowledge your fear. This is where self-awareness is so powerful and has such value.

Self-awareness is a bag of frozen peas.

Confused?

It's the bag of frozen peas that I put on my toe after I stubbed it on my bed. That cool iciness helped me make sense of what was going on in my body. I could finally realize the pain was in my toe, check what happened, and decide whether the toe is broken. This allowed me to reflect on the other sensations in my body, from the aching cramp in my shoulders from almost backflipping onto my mattress when my toe connected with the bed to my fingers cramping from squeezing my foot so tightly for what seemed to be forever.

Your bag of peas could be a quiet afternoon of meditation so you can reflect on what you are feeling after a breakup, following someone you love's funeral, or after some significant loss. Loss is something you go through, and while you feel it too, it's not all you feel.

You can't go on until you deal with those feelings, see them, know them, and acknowledge them. After all, anger is one of the stages of the famous Kübler-Ross grief model. When I applied my personalized bag of frozen peas to my pain, I began to realize resentment, anger, loneliness, fear, sorrow, regret, and a whole range of other emotions that I had been masking with pain. Only once I was aware of these could I begin to know myself, see my path into my future where I could be free from loss, and begin to let go.

This is a process, and it may take several "bags of frozen peas," so be kind to yourself, but do the work required to know and believe in yourself so that you can begin the process of letting go.

UNDERSTANDING YOUR OWN LIMITS

Once I made sense of what I was feeling, I realized that I couldn't do it all alone. I needed help, and there is no shame in asking for or accepting help. While your friends may have offered to "be there for you when you need a shoulder to cry on," this may be too close for you to feel comfortable, or they may be biased. Professional help is not a sign of weakness. By seeing a trained therapist, you are taking care of yourself and not battling it alone so you can continue to take care of others. This self-care is what you may need to help you let go. It's the preparation you require to plant the seeds of your future.

Not everyone wants to go to a therapist or, as had success, so they prefer to help themselves or talk to a friend. I had many friends who were hurting from trauma and death that didn't want to go that route and instead came to me. My limits required that I learn other ways outside of traditional therapies to help myself and move forward. I began a quest to learn how to heal and read extensively within psychotherapy and Holistic practices.

I came across an article where I discovered ways to heal from my childhood trauma and abuse. This freedom from pain was so intriguing that it led to training and becoming a certified NLP practitioner and Life Coach. This path to self-healing helped me reach a stage in my life to help others face their emotions and let go. It became the main driving force, my fire and, my life's purpose on this earth. Helping others has always been my passion and why I found such joy in my career in the medical field. If it weren't for the experiences that I went through, I wouldn't be on this path of helping others heal emotionally or writing this book.

Your journey will look different. Your limits will help you move forward once you know them and make the most of your limitations. With my training, I also understood that boundaries are there to be challenged and improved. This is what happens when you begin to let go of the things that impose limitations on you. You grow, learning from the experience taking with you, not the hurt, but the lesson.

GETTING READY TO LET GO

So, you want to let go? It's not simply something you do one day, like changing your shoes. Instead, when you are beginning to let go, you have to do so thoroughly. That means you need to acknowledge your:

Feelings

Only once you know what you are feeling can you begin to let go.

Limitations

By knowing what is holding you back, you can see the things that tie you down.

Challenges

There are obstacles in your path to self-healing and letting go. Your friends or family may expect you to grieve still or grieve in a way that makes sense to them, which can be a considerable obstacle.

Needs

Once you know what you need to begin healing and letting go, you can start releasing the tension, negative energies, and self-defeating thoughts that stop you from letting go.

Once you are ready to begin letting go, you can take the first steps to release your feelings and learned behavior. Knowing you are ready to let go may require more skills than my story within this first chapter, but you can become prepared to open and release by completing the following action steps.

ACTION STEP 1: ARE YOU READY TO ACCEPT?

Most therapists will tell you to write in a journal or scribble somewhere to let out your feelings. Not everyone likes or wants to write. It's the fear of re-reading what you wrote that might not make any sense, have difficulty getting the words out or, just don't like to write at all. Writing can be both liberating and damning. When I started writing for the first time, I was skeptical and hesitant. I didn't want to write and couldn't see the value in it. What is the purpose of writing down intimate thoughts and feelings like a teenager with a diary? Logically, I knew that I couldn't say out loud most of what I was feeling, and writing that mess down may make me feel better. So, I persevered in my journal, and I can't equate just how valuable the following journal activities were. I am sure they will help you prepare to let go too. Writing them down, getting them out of our heads and hearts assists with the letting go process. What you can't say to someone or that you don't want to say out loud gets put down on paper.

Start by getting a notebook. Try to avoid going for something pretty that you won't want to write your emotions into the pages. It doesn't have to be fancy; even a college notebook will do with a lot of paper. If you're going to weep into your pages, smudging ink, and curling the page corners, then do so and make your writing unapologetic.

Ready?

Emotional Flood

Start by writing down precisely what happened as if you are reporting it to the local news. You may feel like you are about to burst. So, do it. Burst! Let all the feelings spill onto the page. Weep if you must; even if you think you've already cried a river and can't possibly cry more, you can still let the tears spill. While your emotions spill forth, let your pen be busy too. Write anything and everything that comes into your mind. Don't set a time limit on it. Don't worry about grammar, punctuation, or even making sentences; that's not the point. Just write. Draw too, if that helps. Put what you are feeling onto paper, even if it doesn't make sense.

When I did this activity after my son's stillbirth, I spent most of a rainy Saturday afternoon just scribbling, almost filling half a notebook. As a caution: Don't expect to feel better magically. I felt empty once I had written. So incredibly empty and utterly exhausted. I had been carrying the weight of my grief, and only some months after the loss did I finally lay that burden down.

So, I slept a little, had a cup of tea, and finally, I read the tear-soaked pages, deciphering ink blotches and runny writing. It was chaotic, but then I had felt utterly confused and lost, so it was no surprise that my writing would look like that.

While reading, I noticed a pattern emerging. Taking a different color pen, I began to circle certain words or phrases that stood out to me. This was where I started to see that what I felt was so much more than endless pain. It was the self-blame, non-forgiveness, and resentment that I read on those pages. It was the perpetual loss and not wanting to move past. I didn't even know how or where to begin. The writing was also the beginning of my journey to self-healing and forgiveness. I realized during that difficult afternoon that it would start with me, and this was the only place where my healing *could* begin. The hurt underneath was stacked with layers of pain that had me caught in a web of misery. It was acknowledging what I felt and the negative self-talk.

With this realization, I began to understand that I was ready to start loosening my grip on my grief and start to let go. I was prepared to begin my release journey. Perhaps there was something to the saying of "no pain, no gain."

2

IT BEGINS WITH YOU

One may walk over the highest mountain one step at a time.

— BARBARA WALTERS

I t had become my morning routine. I would wake up, lie in bed, and look up at the ceiling fan. The feeling of dead weight on my chest or just not being able to get up would fill me. I used to think, "Oh, my gosh, not another morning." Everything hurt. My body had become a physical expression of my inner state. In clinical terms, this is known as having psychosomatic symptoms. My mind and soul were so tired, but the near-fatal fatigue was expressing itself in my body.

I knew the meaning of being soul-tired.

If this resonates with you, you will likely have an unresolved loss that makes you run away. Carrying the weight of those emotions with you is like having the weight of the world dragging behind you. To make matters worse, you also have others who depend on you. There seems to be no break in sight, no end to your agony. Pretty soon, depression sets in, and you become wrapped up in your pain.

I was a functioning depressive person. This meant that I could hold down a job, take care of my kids, and cook dinner, but I was in agony all the way. I didn't permit myself to lie down and lick my wounds. Perhaps I should have.

So, one fateful day, I was making sub sandwiches for the family when the knife slipped and cut my finger quite badly. Sticking it out and carrying on had become my method, so I quickly put on a band-aid, then I continued with dinner. Several days later, the cut had become infected, and I ended up at the doctor's office.

The wise and older gentlemen at the clinic told me that I was not taking care of the wound, which was why it had gotten worse. As he cleaned out the wound, placed the right medicine on it, and taped it up, I began to have an epiphany: I hadn't been taking care of my soul-wound either. My loss had started, like that cut, to fester. I had to take responsibility and use self-care and self-therapy to help my almost fatal soul-wound to heal.

This chapter is all about you, how you can begin to self-care and use self-therapy.

THE IMPORTANCE OF TAKING A BREAK

"Take a break ... have a Kitkat." I must have eaten a dozen a day at one stage as I tried to comfort myself, and while the candy wasn't a good idea, the slogan was. I needed to take a break. What I realized immediately was that while dramatic examples appeal to us, like taking a road trip for three weeks or going on a cruise, we need those little five-minute breaks too. I'm not saying you need to eat chocolates every couple of minutes, but I am saying you need to take a break every so often.

During the day, having just a few minutes to yourself every so often is a great way to begin self-healing. It's like applying a soothing balm to that cut finger of mine, except it's some me-time for my soul-wound. The doctor had told me to apply the medicine every time the finger ached, to rinse it diligently with a medical wash at least three times a day, and to wrap it up snuggly. I realized this advice was entirely appropriate to my soul-wound too.

I had to take care of myself at least three times a day. When the pain grew too much, I had to rinse my wound with the appropriate self-therapy. If I didn't take care of my soul-wound, I would likely end up suffering an amputation from myself.

What I came to realize is that it's not even something massive I had to do. I just had to take better care of myself. Oh, for sure, it wasn't all success in the beginning. I tried some retail therapy, which didn't help at all. Then I began looking for other ways to numb the pain, but I wasn't doing anything that had been healing myself. I didn't need a seven-day Caribbean cruise or a long road trip to Montana. Instead, I just needed to do something small every day to help me stop, breathe, think, and become peaceful.

The problem was, looking at my pain, I started to feel over-whelmed. I began to doubt that I had the strength to start, much less let go. Only once I began to really look at my soul-wound and actively take steps to sit back and take a break did I begin to heal. So, I made time to have a daily cup of hot tea where I made a little ritual to help me relax and just breathe.

It may sound like it was simple to accomplish. It wasn't. It's was one of the hardest things for me to do. I forced myself to sit and try to keep my body still. Not very simple when you feel like it's still traveling at the speed of light! My brain was also rushing with thoughts, and I would begin to have internal arguments and feel guilty for taking a time-out that I desperately needed. "Just sit still with so much to do? I have a home to keep straight, laundry to wash, fold and put away, and children to care for. I don't have time for 'me time!'" Perhaps this resonates with you as well and, that's just it. You will have to *make* "me time" just as I did because you deserve to have a period of inner focus and quiet. It may be challenging to accomplish, but it's necessary.

I would get out my favorite teacup and saucer design that my momma gave to me. Staffordshire made it exclusively for Avon in the 1970s. Every time I used it, I always felt so content and calm. I would sit on the sofa by the window in silence or, sometimes, with a book ready for me to read. I would sip as I allowed myself to relax and be in the moment. This was my "medical wash" for my soul-wound, and soon, the infection in my soul began to draw out, and I began to heal.

When I ran across meditation, I felt a load lift off me that focused on breathing and visualization. If being able to visu-alize is difficult for you to achieve, then solely focus on the breathing part of this exercise. This tool can be applied anytime you feel stressed, not only for your five-minute break. I use this technique often during life stresses. It's in the same line as counting to ten widely used, where you're only focusing on the counting. This technique alone effectively assists you in letting go of the stress that can cause health issues.

Stress triggers high cortisol levels to be released from the adrenal gland. These levels result in high glucose (blood sugar), numerous health issues such as high blood pressure, depression, digestive problems, anxiety, and more. Chronic stress is commonly known as a "silent killer," and why many therapists suggest stress-reducing techniques such as visualization and breathing exercises.

To begin this exercise, I would sit with my cup of tea, eyes closed, and visualize that the air I breathed in was positive bright healing air. Then, I would hold it to the count of five, seeing the light flowed into my lungs, then spreading to every part of my body. As I exhaled, I saw the air flowing out of me as dark pent-up smoke. I repeated this exercise until I felt calm, usually no less than two minutes. These breathing and visualizing techniques were and are powerful tools in my recovery toolbox. Seeing the stress leaving my body unleashed a flood of calm in my mind and made me feel energized and lowered my pulse.

It wasn't important what I chose to do in my five-minute break, but it did matter that I took one. Taking a break meant I could shift my perspective, and in doing so, I could see things differently without being so stressed. I could consider solutions to my daily problems that previously had me unable even to think. I found that things didn't seem quite so bad after that bit of breathing and a cup of English tea.

Your five-minute breaks could look a bit differently from mine that was shrouded in nostalgia. You could walk in your garden, play with your kids or dogs for a bit, listen to music, or sit in silence. Whatever you decide to use as a break, make sure you take some time off and just relax. Like the famous tagline from a well-known hair color brand, it's "because you're worth it."

THE BENEFITS OF AN OPEN MIND

Part of healing is to develop an open mind. Pain can leave us closed off to those around us, and only when we open our minds can we begin to accept others and ourselves. When I started to deal with my pain, I struggled to understand why bad things happen and why I couldn't move on. This was because my mind focused on the pain. I wasn't open-minded enough to consider all aspects of my pain and the tragic incidents that had steered me into suffering.

I needed to cultivate an open mind. Being open-minded helped me see things from a different perspective and come up with answers to painful questions. New ideas and thoughts meant I could begin to find new medicines for my soul wound. An open mind helped me think rationally (Cherry, 2021).

By cultivating an open mind, I:

Could Listen to Others

Before, when I was locked in my own perspective of my pain, I couldn't hear people out when they seemed to have a different opinion about my loss. While I welcomed sympathy, I couldn't stand it either. I needed empathy, but I almost zealously guarded my pain and wouldn't let others share it. Once I started developing an open mind, I could let people into my circle.

Could Empathize With Others

Pain is usually not something we experience in isolation, and by being open-minded, I could start to understand what others were feeling in their heads. That helped me feel a sense of connection. Being an empath, I could *feel* their emotions, but they sometimes didn't match their thoughts.

Experienced Personal Growth

Open-mindedness means you can see yourself in a new light, and you can use this different perspective to create new insights and stimulate personal growth. Removing negative self-talk will assist in being more open-minded. That inner voice change will also allow you to visualize a better self.

Grew Stronger and More Agile in My Mind

Grief is stressful, and when you feel stressed over the long term, your brain chemistry goes all out of whack from the high cortisol levels previously covered. You can't think straight, feel panicked in a "fight or flight" sort of way, and all you can focus on is your pain. Embracing mindfulness decreases your stress levels, and soon, you will begin to experience a sense of calm, which leads to clarity of thought and a more agile mind.

Consider Other Elements of an Open Mind

When you practice having an open mind, you will become more positive, not easy, I know, so it takes some practice, and you will be less self-absorbed. That means you stop wallowing in your misery and actively begin doing things that help you feel better. You move from victimhood to being an active participant in your life again. Your pain no longer owns you, and you can take ownership of your pain so you can manage it, resolve it, and begin to heal emotionally.

LOOKING INWARDS AND HAVING A QUIET SURROUNDING

I discovered that while I struggled through my grief and loss, the mind becomes a meat grinder. Everything churns, and the stress burns your nerve endings, causing pain and numbness. The best cure for anxiety is a peaceful environment and peaceful introspection. When you reflect on your worries and pain, you can assign value to these realistically and logically. This helps you cope and adjust to your burden.

Having a quiet surrounding environment will significantly help you reduce the internal noise that churns through your mind. Like someone with post-traumatic stress disorder (PTSD), you would do well in environments that are soothing with no sudden noises or disturbances. This may also mean that you don't need people to crowd your spaces. You may require some solitude to clear your mind and quiet the chaos inside. Being a sufferer diagnosed with Complex PTSD at that time, I found this to be effective.

Be careful about not indulging in complete long periods of isolation as it is not healthy. You may think that it would be best for everyone for you to just deal with it alone; it isn't.

Avoid this type of reasoning at all costs. Isolating yourself surrounds you with walls of pain that echo loudly like a migraine that intensifies. Balancing quiet time with being around other people will limit the frustrations you are experiencing as it preserves your inner light.

A good analogy is that you have a lit candle shining with a big flame within you at the start of every day. This flame represents your inner light, peace, and energy. Life, emotions, and people naturally take some of the light throughout the day without lowering the height of the fire and snuffing it out. But when all you do is focus on your pain, the flame starts to stifle out until the candle barely flickers. You haven't the energy to focus on anything else in life that needs tending. You've used all or majority of your light in being submerged in your pain and loss. To counter this from occurring, have moments of quiet solitude to quiet your mind. It will help you rebalance and recharge so that you can be around loved ones and friends. If you find moments where you need to shut yourself inside of your closet to have five minutes of peace, then do so. Be careful not to cut out your family or loved ones for support. You need them just as much as they need you. Sometimes, you just need time to be. This is one of the first steps you need to take: finding peace around you so you can find and create harmony within.

ONE STEP AT A TIME

Following each of the incidents of loss I had suffered, I wanted to run away. I tried to rush forward, just get moving, and somehow just forget about the pain I felt and bury it. However, I realized that a journey begins with one step, and when you are ready, you can take another and another. You don't start sprinting even if it feels scary at times.

I had to teach myself only to take one step at a time and not rush ahead. I had to focus mentally and emotionally on healing each aspect then move one step. I had to settle on that initiative or that moment. While I wanted to run away from the grief, I had to address it entirely, which I knew would take time. As the saying goes, "Rome wasn't built in a day." There's no point in lying about it: the pain of moving so slowly towards my recovery was excruciating. But I was building a firm foundation and a clear mind to carry me forward to healing. It would be like building a house on sand, expecting it to hold up under pressure without doing this. Rushing might seem quicker, but it would only take longer to get there in the end.

When you move slowly and deliberately through pain, you can begin to see the lessons that abound, and you can learn from your loss. This is how healing works: you need to learn, grow, and move on. It all begins with one step, and you need to move slowly, experiencing each moment so you can have the opportunity to learn and grow.

DEVELOPING EMOTIONAL FLOW

Your emotions express your energies, and when you block your feelings, you lose the power to step forward. To avoid this, you need to develop emotional flow. This means you need to acknowledge all emotions, yes, the bad ones too. You are angry for the loss you have suffered, as well you are also saddened by this. Feel it. Don't turn away or avoid looking at the negative things you feel. Don't judge these feelings, and refrain from seeing them as being bad or shameful. Accept that as a whole human, you are entitled to feel the full spectrum of emotions.

Only when you let yourself feel everything can you begin to heal. What you have been classifying as being in pain may be a range of feelings, from anger and betrayal at being left behind by the one you lost to regret at not having had the time to say what you needed to say. Once these emotions have had the time to flow through you, it will become less challenging to admit your feelings.

Negative emotions are like children who are naughty and ignored. You need to acknowledge them. By listening to them and hearing them out, you can settle them down. Finally, you will have a chance at peace of mind.

Using your journal to write about your feelings that are hard to talk about is a great way to settle them, turn them over, and take charge of yourself. Grief must run its course. Your emotions need to run their course too. Open the floodgates, let those feelings you don't want to show others cascade out until you are run empty of feeling. Then you can begin to heal. I've often compared this to this visual. All of the negative thoughts and emotions are dark clouds that build up inside, and once they have gathered, it's a storm with either rain or rage that emerges. Let go of the dark clouds within you. You'll feel better once you do!

When your emotions have run out, you can begin to live and focus on the present. If your focus is on this moment right now, you are stepping beyond grief, which is in the past. You are also letting go of the anguish of loss that echoes into the future. No, you won't get to be with that person you loved again in the future. However, you are here, right now, and you can live here in this moment, and then in the next moment.

PERMISSION TO LET GO

When your emotions have settled, you reach the point where you can permit yourself to let go. For me, that point only came a few years after the loss of my stillborn son. After his death, I had conceived two daughters without any difficulties. But I carried the rage, regret, and depression with me for a long time after his death. It was only once I delved into self-healing and NLP practices that I began to realize that letting go was more than a decision. It was about permitting myself to let go.

If you are unsure what this means for you, then read the following permission statements aloud and notice how they make you feel:

- I can live freely now, and I permit myself to let go of all the things that have been weighing me down.
- I allow myself to live in this moment, let go of the past, and prepare with hope for the future.
- My permission to move on is something I give myself freely as I don't need suffering anymore.
- I forgive myself, and I let go of regrets because I need to move forward.

I still feel tears in my eyes when I read these for my former self and all that I was enduring. They become like rays of light that shine into my inner darkness, melting the icy fortress I had built around my pain. I was permitting myself to be free. With these acceptance and permission statements, I was saying to myself the words I had not wanted to listen to from others: "It's okay. You will be okay."

Accepting that I could let go was a significant deal for me! It should be that big for you too. However, as you may notice, you are only a quarter of a way through this book, and your journey to self-forgiveness, healing, and letting go is just starting. Permitting yourself, taking things one step at a time, and releasing your emotions are only the beginning. There is still much work to be done in your journey of letting go and returning to yourself.

ACTION STEP 2: ARE YOU READY TO LET GO?

Time to pull the journal closer. In Chapter 1, you wrote about your feelings, your deep and painful experience of your grief, and now it's time to write about your first efforts at surviving and demolishing it. Even though you may not want to write, getting into a routine will help you. I understand that you may not want to do this activity because you're hurting so badly. Writing your feelings and emotions out can help you heal. Writing about the pain you felt is the medicine, and the steps you're taking towards the cure are the bandaids. I know it hurts, and I understand your objections to not writing them out, or you don't know how to start. Perhaps not making the whole pot of coffee that you did for you both to feel as if they are there, or blocking the person on your phone so that you don't keep checking to see if they've messaged or called. Making a plan to combat your loss can assist you in the steps of healing because you've acknowledged and listed your game plan to moving forward.

Use your journal with each of the activities of this chapter. When you take some time off to be alone and sit in silence, keep your journal near. You may not always want to write in it, but having it there is a gentle reminder that you can use the time for a few lines as you slowly draw out the pain of your loss. Your journal is part of your recovery toolkit—a place where you can pour your emotions into instead of keeping them locked deep inside or, worse, thrown like daggers at those around you. Trying to suppress your feelings will only serve to intensify them later.

I remember writing a journal entry many years after my father died. While much of it is so profoundly personal and chaotic that it would make no sense to someone other than myself, I do want to share a section here from several years ago. It was a day of remembrance and a very emotional one that was a turning point in my healing. Perhaps you can relate to it:

My daddy died. It's not recent, but it's still so raw. He left my life a long time ago, which I resented. How I could have used daddy's words of advice when I was living my life, making my choices, but instead, he died.

I still feel resentment that he broke up our family, and though his death anniversary was now almost 12 years ago, I still struggle. How do I let go? Why can't I even speak all of the words I wanted to say to him, not just that I forgave him? I dread birthdays. Now so does my daughter. He was diagnosed on my birthday and then buried on hers. His prognosis was two years that turned into being two days. Why didn't the doctors figure his illness out sooner?! I still had a leftover birthday cake in the fridge from my daughter's 13th birthday. How bizarre that the day of mine and my daughter's birth were now so closely intertwined with his death and burial. My baby girl officially became a teenager on the day of his funeral. I cry for her sake too. She lost her papa, and I lost my daddy. I should have been consoling my stepmother, but instead, I was a complete wreck. I sobbed uncontrollably throughout the service, and then at his graveside, I laid down a single red rose with my goodbye as I hugged his coffin, refusing to let go. I finally said the words he'd begged me for, but I was just too late, "daddy, I forgive you!" As he was buried, so did I with my grief and regrets.

Will I be in mourning forever?

How can I get over this pain that is consuming me? What do I need to do to take steps forward for all I have bottled up for 12 years? It won't stay buried no matter how hard I try; it just keeps rising up! I'm tired of crying on our birthdays each year. It should be a happy time with the family, instead, I dwell in the past with my deceased father. This year will be different. It has to be. This year, no matter how hard it is to do this, I will allow myself to let go. Daddy, I love and miss you so much! You're dying will never be okay, but I am okay. I am much stronger than this grief and regret, and I need to let go of this pain and sorrow. I can't continue doing this every year, it's killing me! I'm missing out on so much. I'm still here, and so are your three granddaughters. It's time to make a change. I have to for our sake and live for the future instead of for your death in the past.

Reading this passage puts into perspective the amount of suffering I endured and the pain I put myself through. My regret for not giving my father the absolution that he'd begged for, mingled with hating myself for making him suffer, locked me into a dark tower of grief. The saddest words to ever hear is "it's too late." My regrets kept me from freedom and locked within my tower of grief. Acceptance and forgiveness were the keys to my release and, only after I acknowledged what I couldn't change and forgive did I begin to heal and live again.

What will your journal entries look like? Have you locked yourself into the tower holding your heart and life hostage? Write about the pain and let the pages capture the bitterness, resentment, and anger from your tower of grief. When you are ready, begin to look for that moment of slowly letting go. As the door swings open, you'll find that you are free and able to leave that place. You will realize that you are ready to change and walk out of the tower once you accept and give forgiveness. Then, you are prepared to let go.

3

MAKE A CHANGE

If you change the way you look at things, the things you look at change.

— WAYNE DYER

I read a book on habit formation, and like so many of these books, it contained such exciting insights. However, what really stuck with me was the bit about replacing a bad habit instead of trying to stop it. I had a lightbulb moment!

To let go of something meant I had to replace it with a more positive experience. Simply deciding to let go of something wouldn't help, as this meant I would have a void in my life.

Where I had been defining myself by my pain, I needed to redefine myself based on something else. To let go requires change.

It would be painful. I won't lie to you. But in the end, it was worth it for me, and as you'll see, it will be worth it for you. I discovered that if I changed the things I looked at, I could change the way things looked to me. I could find hope by stopping my own regurgitated feasting on my loss. It was all about perspective and using it to assist in the process of the loss.

This chapter will share a few things I found while I processed my grief and began to look forward to new and different things.

WHY TEARS HELP

In the beginning, I cried because I was hurt. I sensed the losses I suffered in a very personal and painful way. It would be unnatural not to cry following the death of a parent or the loss of your child. I even wept during my divorce at times. Weeping is normal. Most people won't challenge you on crying during a funeral or weeks later, but why did I still keep on sobbing many years later when the death anniversary of my dad's passing rolled around? That was something people did begin to question. It was challenging to deal with, and my family was confused by the unstoppable weeping I still experienced every year around my birthday. Even 12 years after his passing, I still cried as if he had just died today! Why?

This led me to start researching why we cry. I found some interesting studies, with one in particular by Dr. William Frey II, who conducted research at Ramsey Medical Center in Minneapolis, which touched me. His research confirmed my theory that crying was actually a coping mechanism of your body (Deschene, n.d.).

So, when you cry, there are two reasons to do this. Firstly, as you know, we get reflex tears that lubricate and protect our eyes. Secondly, and most importantly, we get emotional tears. Researchers have analyzed these tears, and they discovered that the tears contained harmful hormones and chemicals that are known to trigger the release of our body's natural stress hormone (cortisol). So, by crying, you flush these harmful chemicals to prevent your stress levels from increasing. Your body is protecting itself, as we all know that stress is a killer. Therefore, crying reduces stress (Mann, 2011). How intriguing!

When I began weeping each year on daddy's death anniversary, I was protecting myself. My tears were flushing away chemicals that could have caused me great harm. That also meant I felt better after crying. My advice to you is to let yourself cry. And cry as often as you need it. Your body can't always consciously tell you what is happening with your chemical mix, so you may be needing those tears to release stress and pain. By not crying, you are increasing your stress and suffering.

If you are struggling with crying, which I have seen in some of the lovely people I have counseled for grief, you need to find ways to start crying. Perhaps ask a few good friends over while you unpack your dearly departed person's belongings? Maybe kick back with a few tear-jerker movies to help lubricate your eyes and purge your emotions? Don't tell yourself myths such as "you need to be strong for your children, don't let them see you cry" or "crying won't bring him back, so don't waste your tears." I've done that, and it doesn't work. Crying is natural and a way to get past a difficult situation.

Let your body and mind weep as much as you need, and give yourself the gift of time to do your crying.

THE POWER OF YOUR FOCUS

God, grant me the serenity to accept the things I cannot change and the courage to change the things I can. And the wisdom to know the difference.

— REINHOLD NIEBUHR, THE
SERENITY PRAYER

This first verse of the venerable Serenity Prayer has always lingered in my mind. A friend gifted me with a plaque engraved with this, and when I look at it, I am reminded that we can choose on which to focus. It may be quite a mind shift to think like this, but it is possible. Yes, it's terrible to lose someone, and there's nothing you can do to bring that person back, but instead of thinking, "why me?" begin to think, "what can I learn from this?"

You have the power to refocus your mind, your intention, and your energies. Instead of focusing on the loss, focus on what has changed for the better or what you have learned. There is always something beneficial if you look hard enough.

What can you change? Yes, you are suffering your loss, but what can you change? Can you choose to look at the experience in a different light?

When you start cultivating this kind of thinking, you are sure to start watering the roots of change, as I did. As a word of warning, your inner self may scream and rebel against this mind shift. After all, how could anything positive come from your tragedy? Remember, it's not about saying the loss was good. It's about looking for some silver lining to a dark event or tragedy. If you look hard enough, you will find something. Something such as losing someone reignited a relationship with a family member or a friend that if it weren't for your loss, the renewed relationship would not have happened.

Perhaps a breakup made you look at your appearance or health, and you decided to eat better and become healthier. That is a positive out of a negative situation. We sometimes get into a rut and tend not to focus inward as much as we probably should.

Losing my daddy, who was only 62 years old so quickly, was an obvious negative. The positive was that it made me more aware that life can be cut short and cherish my momma more. They are just as vulnerable as you and I are, regardless of how tough and bulletproof we made them out to be.

OPENING UP ROOM TO CHANGE

Years ago, an Oprah show where some celebrity home fixer was busy talking about how you need to throw out your old clothes to open up room for the new ones. While this may have been practically intended, I still recall the idea of throwing out old things to have new things come into your life.

This ties in with the law of attraction, which has so many followers worldwide. The basic tenet is that what you put out, you attract; when you throw out to make space, you will welcome in things you need. Holding onto something that no longer serves you will block the flow of energy, and you will be stuck with a loss instead of opening up to new and beautiful things.

When you are grieving a loss, this can be difficult to do. How do you let go of the person you lost and hope you will find something good to replace them? But that's just it: I discovered it's not the person you lost you are throwing out. It's simply the pain of the loss of them that you have to let go.

I have chosen to let go of the painful two days my father was ill before his death. I choose to focus on the life he had with me. By recalling fond memories I have of him, such as watching him play guitar while he sang or rehearsing for the gospel quartet he was in, I can still value his life. However, I let go of his death. I choose not to let his dying and eventual death overshadow his life. He was much more than his demise. By not clinging to my regrets about what I wanted to say to him but couldn't, I can open myself to new experiences and the joy of living. I couldn't let his death define him, and as harsh as this may sound, I couldn't allow it to define me either.

What can you let go of in your journey with loss? What can you welcome into your life when you begin to create space for change?

CUTTING OUT THE HURT TO BRING HEALING

Clinging to hurt is like closing up a wound before you have cleaned it. The infection spreads inward with nowhere to go, eating away at your flesh and making a larger wound. Like that cut on my finger that I hadn't looked after, it needs some serious cleaning out before the healing can begin. The doctor had to surgically cut little bits of my finger away to leave healthy tissue to grow and heal the injury. He cut the hurt away. How can you cut the pain away?

Whatever your loss is, it has been in your life for a long time. You've been holding onto it for many months or years, so as a result, the pain has eaten into your soul, leaving a much bigger wound that is not healing. Learning to let go of pain and welcoming change is a way to clean out that wound; cutting away the infected soul tissue allows the healing to begin.

For me, I combined this with the realization that I had to replace that pain with something healthy. I had to find ways to occupy my time where I previously had been absorbed with my loss and tragedy. Memories of the loss were replaced by fond, joyful thoughts about the person who passed. Even my husband, who moved on after our divorce, could be celebrated for the good times we had together (even though there were terrible times within). The positive; he gave me three beautiful daughters that I would repeatedly endure every bit of it just to have them.

Instead of spending time contemplating painful memories, I could go out and seek to live in the now. I began singing more often, writing poems, watched movies, and spent time with my three daughters. Slowly, once I had removed the pain, I began to heal and live again. This would not have been possible without first letting go. I had to let go of several things, including my anger, negativity, and sorrow.

LETTING GO OF ANGER

I realized that anger was beginning to consume me. It was like gangrene, eating through my body and my soul. I had to amputate my rage. It was probably one of the most painful things to do. I remember writing and writing in my journal, bleeding onto the page until I had cleaned all the rage and was left empty of hate.

Firstly, I had to really feel my anger. I had to let myself know who and towards what directed my anger. I had to fix what was bleeding before I bled on those who didn't cut me. By clinging to my anger, I was bleeding on those who were still alive and with me: my daughters and my family.

I raged. There were days when I drove down the highway belting out my lungs to the loudest music I could find, thoroughly purging my anger. Finally, I began to accept the anger, letting it slowly dribble away. And I began to heal.

Physical activities helped. Getting out into nature or at the ocean soothed me, and dancing freed me. I began to look at the beautiful things in my life, and these filled up the empty wound space I had been left with once my anger was purged.

RELEASING NEGATIVE FEELINGS

With the time spent on my loss and anger, I had built up a floodgate that had kept all my negative feelings in check. I needed to let these go, so I had to begin to release the pressure. By searching for answers, I found a range of techniques that helped me with this task. None of these were quick fixes. Instead, they were treatments to help me heal, and I still use many of them today as side companions to NLP techniques to keep me balanced and focused on the positive in life.

Finding Joy

By finding new and exciting things to invest my time in, I could replace frustration with joy. I could learn new skills, take up new hobbies, and find ways to draw positive energy into my life. Before I started something new, I would ask myself: Is this good for me?

Finding Peace

Each step I took forward had to bring me some measure of peace. If it was going to give me stress, then I chose not to walk in that direction. So, I began to focus on mindfulness while I meditated and did yoga. I went for long walks, and I read inspirational stories. I reconnected with family I had been neglecting, and I spent hours alone, simply content to be in my own company.

I began to live more positively. That meant consciously and subconsciously helping my mind to look for opportunities. When I started to drift back into my old and negative thinking patterns, I would replace this with positive thoughts. I would find myself wondering why I had to lose my unborn son. I could feel the anger rise in my throat, threatening to choke me; however, I countered these thoughts by telling myself that I had been given two beautiful daughters after his death that I wouldn't have had who are here with me. I can be all I am with them, living a life of joy. There is no place for anger where joy and peace exist.

Develop a New Narrative

We all have our stories that we tell ourselves and others. This is how you see your life as unfolding. I focused on the tragedy that filled my life, which became the central feature in my personal story. I had created a narrative around these. Yet, my life was filled with so many other amazing people and events. By choosing to focus on these, I could start creating a new narrative. I could make up my life story in a positive and meaningful way. Death and loss no longer needed to be the central theme of my life.

Forgive and Stop Blaming

When something terrible happens, we are quick to blame. When my son died, I looked for someone to blame. Were the doctors at fault? Was my body responsible? Had I done something during the pregnancy that had somehow contributed to his stillbirth? I wanted to blame someone and finding nobody else. I began to blame myself. Have you reached this point? Did you also try blaming others and finally ended up blaming yourself?

I'm here to tell you that it wasn't your fault. You are not to blame for the loss you suffered. Even if you did something to precipitate the loss of someone you love, you might not have known better at that time, and you know better now. You don't have to shoulder the blame for the rest of your life. That wouldn't be fair, and you can forgive yourself. Regret and "If only" can and will haunt you, so once you forgive yourself, you can let that go as well.

Most religions of the world promulgate the idea of forgiving others and finding forgiveness for yourself. You can seek forgiveness, make atonement, and you can let go of the blame. There is no need for your life to end with the loss. By continuing to feel the loss and wearing it like some badge of honor, you simply add yourself to the list of the walking dead. You stroll around, but your loss has stopped you from living because of being frozen in that time, unable to move forward. We are either busy living or busy dying. I know which I chose. It's time for you also to get busy living again.

Change can be painful, and it's not an easy or fast process, but it is worth it. You are worth it! Your family is worth it! Start to let go, embrace change, and seek to live each day, honoring the loss you have suffered but no longer letting it weigh you down.

ACTION STEP 3: ARE YOU READY TO CHANGE?

Using your journal, you can also begin to change. You may not want to write about it, but removing your pain is essential, and writing is the simplest way to move the emotions from within yourself. You can start to notice when you are ready to move on. You may choose to spill all of your anger and rage onto the pages, but you can also use your journal to reflect on the following questions. They will tell you whether you're stuck in your loss or if you are becoming ready to move ahead.

- Do you still wonder about what could have been, or do you look to the future (or even think of tomorrow or next week)?
- Have you begun to think of yourself and the people who are in your life now? Or do you still think

about the person you lost almost every waking moment of your life?

- Do you talk less about the person who died or left, or do you mention them less and less in your conversations?
- When you feel low, do you wish the person you lost was still there to talk to, or do you find someone close to you whom you can turn?

While you may feel ready to change, you should remember that change is a gradual step. It's not a leap of faith. You don't wake up one morning feeling all better and changed. Instead, it's like walking through oil. You take a step or two forward to slide back half or more each time. Keep going. You can and will get there as long as you can stop negative behaviors and replace them with positive ones.

4

STOP WHAT YOU'RE DOING

Your grief path is yours alone, and no one else can walk it, and no one else can understand it.

— TERRI IRWIN

When you have suffered any substantial loss, you realize you are floating in one spot. You know you should let go and move on, but you are stuck there in limbo, unable to head into the rest of your life. Desperate to hold onto the person you lost, you create a shrine for them in your life.

After my unborn son's death, I recall that I struggled for the longest time to let go of the blue boy sleepers and clothes in his baby room. How I longed to see his tiny shape lying in the crib or wiggling in the bassinet. But it wasn't meant to be.

When I walked down the street and saw parents with their newborns, I would become weepy, even months after I had miscarried. Yet, I still looked for things related to a new baby boy. Despite the torture, I would look at newborn clothes, shoes, and toys and think of baby names my husband had considered before we decided on Brandon Christopher. I felt such emptiness, and while I still survived, I felt utterly defeated by the loss and unable to let go. Even after conceiving my second daughter several months later, I clung to Brandon's memory. It wasn't to minimize her at all because I was grateful to be carrying her. The badge of loss was still on my sleeve, and another child isn't a replacement for one lost.

After years of searching and reflection, I finally realized that I had to find a way to move forward and live again. My life couldn't be a shrine to the deceased. Their lives had ended; mine hadn't. Even though their passing was grossly unfair, and I would have given anything to change it, I had to let go and find a way to live with my grief without letting it define me. Yes, it was difficult letting the suffering go, but I had living children that needed their mother just as much as I needed them.

Even when I suffered a loss that wasn't due to death, I still felt myself continuing to hold on. For example, after my divorce, I took the longest time to move forward in my life and just live again. If you believe this isn't true for you, just open your pantry door. Notice how many products there are not there because you like them but rather because your lost person did. You may even continue shopping for things the person who is no longer in your life enjoys long after they have left.

Truly letting go and finding the guts (it does take them) to heal can't happen while focusing on the other person or the past. While you are still holding on to them, nothing else can come into your life. To counter this, you can create a policy of "instead of." This means that instead of buying that product because the person who is no longer there liked it, you will buy something different. Instead of saving space in your home or life for the person who left or passed, you will create space for yourself. And instead of feeling sad, you will feel happy. While swapping sorrow for happiness is a lot more complex than choosing peanut butter over Nutella, this chapter is about finding and celebrating "instead ofs" to help you let go. In doing so, to assist you further into the process and help you find joy and yourself again.

INSTEAD OF THIS, TRY THAT

There are probably many things you think you should be doing when grieving to be free and move on. You may even mentally be preparing yourself for the horrible process of throwing the person you lost out of your life, like last week's newspaper. However, grieving, like life, is about celebration and loss. So instead of focusing on the loss, you should look to the celebration.

When I was searching for my way forward, I read widely. I read all sorts of books on loss and grief while searching for a way through my pain. While more traditional cultures worldwide have rituals, beliefs, and customs to help them process what came after the death of a loved one, our more modern society is somewhat lacking in this aspect. How do we mourn, and how do we move on? What do we have to do after someone's passing from our lives, either through death or a relationship ending?

Out of Sight, Out of Mind

What you're about to read may seem terrible, but when you are already struggling to process the loss of someone from your life, you don't need constant reminders of what you no longer have. There comes a time when you need to begin clearing out your visual space. When you have taken down photos, unfriended, or blocked the person who moved out on social media and started clearing out their stuff, you can open up your heart and mind to new things. This happens because you are no longer wasting energy on rumination over what could have been. Instead, accept what was good when you were with the person who left, and likewise, admit they have moved forward with their lives. You can do this as well because you need to do this for yourself.

It may be more difficult to do when you have lost the person to death. Taking down photos, closing up your parent's or loved one's Facebook account, or turning off reminders of them on social media is heartbreaking, but it is necessary. You can't move on when reminded of all you lost constantly. By extension, this includes removing your loved one's clothes and belongings after they have died.

I recall how many times I sat weeping bitterly in the baby room after my loss. It felt like sacrilege to even think of moving any of the new baby items. But there came the point where I had to do it. I had to release the pain to open up that space and my heart to new possibilities. That is what healing is all about. It's not about forgetting the person who passed; it's about celebrating their life by not letting their death be your only memory of them. It's about making new memories.

My moment of letting go of my son's space in my home came on a lonely afternoon when I was again sitting in his room on the floor, crying and feeling utterly betrayed by God, doctors, and the fates. I started rocking back and forth with my arms across myself, feeling the loss of him like it was brand new. I opened my eyes just as the sun broke through the window shades, lighting up the crib so brightly that it caught me by surprise. There was a feeling of peace that filled me, and I knew it was time. It was as if that was a sign from above that he was watching and that it was ok to move forward. Although it took time to let the sadness go, my acceptance was a start. After four years of trying with Brandon, we conceived our second child shortly after, then our third that following year. What was taken, I was blessed with two-fold.

Your moment of letting go of the things your loved one left behind may not be the same. But at some point, you will know it's time to clear out closets, sell old cars, pack away the personalized stationery you no longer need. Leaving photos of the memories and your loved ones' items will be a constant reminder. Many people get stuck and leave everything undisturbed. It would be better to pack the items you want to keep safely away until you've healed enough to have those reminders.

You might take a few moments to recall adventures that happened at the time of a particular photo, or you could remember how your husband looked in the leather jacket you had bought him. Even though you know you won't be seeing him in that jacket or go on that adventure with him again, you can now let go. You can choose to stop thinking of the loss and start thinking of the possibilities going forward. You can make new memories and take photos of those, and you can let other people enter your life instead of holding out for the one who left.

Use Distance

There is the expression to put some distance between yourself and something painful. This doesn't refer to any actual distance, but that may help too. Going through a divorce, moving to a different house, a new neighborhood, or another city may be what you need to begin the letting process. The same may hold true for more traumatic losses, where being in the space you shared with the person you lost can be too painful for you to be able to let go.

In psychological terms, giving yourself some distance also applies to mentally distancing yourself from the person you have lost. Divorce is not just a legal process. Losing someone to separation or divorce is often also eased by mentally creating some distance by no longer being the wife, husband, or partner as you were before. In other instances, you will need to begin only thinking of yourself as being "you," regaining your true identity, not the role you played. This may be incredibly difficult to do but will give you a little breathing space. Finding yourself as an individual again will assist you in regaining your control into self-discovery.

Use a Mantra, Instead of Ruminating

Losing someone is a little like losing a tooth. You know, that nasty experience where your tongue keeps poking in the hole. Even though you know that you'll get a replacement tooth or denture or grow your adult teeth (if you're a kid), your tongue keeps inspecting the site of damage and loss. When you lose someone, your brain takes on that role. It keeps poking into the area of damage, reminding you constantly of how you feel, what or who you lost, and generally leaving an unpleasant sensation behind. It's that longing for what was or what we had.

When you find your mind poking at the "hole," you can consciously pull it back by using a mantra to stop the rumination. You can use something like:

I loved this person, but I accept they have moved on.
My loss doesn't define me, and I have the power to let go.
I am becoming a whole person following my loss, and I step forward without looking back.
I have always been complete, and this person was a compliment to my wholeness.

Mantras help you change the intensity and type of energy your mind projects. You can decide to alter negative ruminations into positive thoughts that stimulate growth.

Work on Yourself, Instead of Looking at the Other Person

Letting go can also mean you need to release anger and resentment. Instead of focusing on the other person's sins (like in a divorce) or recalling their absence (as in death), you can work on yourself. Who are you now? Take the anger and resentment and transmute them into something positive. Focus on you and not on the other person. Your thinking can change:

Think ...	Instead of ...
→ I am a good person who has a bright future ahead of me.	→ I am alone since my life partner chose to leave me.
→ I can have a life with children and a loving home.	→ This life I lost will never be replaced, and I am broken.
→ My future is within my grasp, and there are so many possibilities ahead of me.	→ Losing this person has left me with nothing, and I don't know how to continue without them.

Live Now, and Not Then

The past is where pain lives. When you linger in the past and contemplate, you will suffer deeply. However, when you live in the present, you can't feel pain or sorrow. Live now, and not then. In this present moment, there is only potential and power. You let go of the agonies of the past and the worries of the future.

Let It Out, Instead of Holding On

When you are trying to let go, it becomes a bad habit to hold onto pain, lock the feelings in place, and stop the energy flow. Feeling the pain isn't pleasant, but you can't lock it away and bury it. Instead, let go and allow the energies to flow through you until equilibrium returns. This is how you get your groove back.

Talk About It, Instead of Keeping Silent

One sad and desperate weekend, my friend lost her boyfriend, who walked away. She was heartbroken and utterly filled with despair. At first, she didn't want to talk about it. She felt betrayed, and she struggled to let go of the pain. Then, she pulled the plug and allowed the pain to purge. Talking does that. It's why we go to psychologists and pay large wads of money while they listen to us during "talk therapy" until our grief has run its course.

Talk about it, and don't keep silent. Speak out instead of letting the words fail you. Part of talking about things is to avoid staying apart from those who would help you. You are not alone.

AVOID SELF-ISOLATION

When you have lost so much, it becomes difficult to open up again. Like a puppy that's been kicked too many times, you are hesitant to trust again and let anyone in. This can lead to self-isolation. Yet, being alone and being on your own is not the same thing.

Sometimes, you need to be on your own. You may need some quiet time with no expectations to conform to and space to engage in self-discovery. Within doing this, it can help you with the final steps of letting go. However, if you choose to be alone because you are afraid, then being alone is not healthy. Being on your own because you don't trust other people or fear you will suffer loss again is like drowning instead of learning to swim.

Self-isolation, when you do so because of fear, is unhealthy and will only increase your pain. It is not about hiding; it's about living. Life doesn't have to stop with you because you're hurting.

Perhaps you are already at this point. Take a moment and think about your behavior in dealing with your pain. Do you skip doing the things that you love to do and stay inside? Do you say no when people ask you to join them in a time out somewhere to have some fun? Do you feel that you haven't the strength to even get through the day? Here's that phrase that I said I would repeat. You are stronger than you give yourself credit. You endured hardships before and were able to move forward and live. Have patience with yourself as you work through your emotions.

THE POWER OF KEEPING BUSY

Being busy can give meaning to your life, even when it feels as if your life has ended. Involve yourself in tasks that occupy your mind, so you don't have time for overthinking. Yes, there will be sad moments, but you will be less inclined to idle and get stuck when you have a reason to get to the other side. Balance being busy by setting aside time for remembering and grieving. You can "schedule" grief for a time more suitable such as in the evening once you've finished the day. Getting your life back to regular routines may sound cold or too logical, it can assist you in feeling normal. Even though you don't feel like going out or working on the hobby you used to enjoy before the loss, doing those things will help you feel normal. You're still here even though they are not.

It is possible to set aside a time of the day for remembrance. That doesn't mean your grief isn't real. It just means you acknowledge that your grief doesn't dominate your life. By knowing there is also time for other things that are meaningful and important, you learn how to balance your life and find your feet. Yes, you are grieving, but you also need to go shopping for toilet paper and milk, take your kids to school, shower, clean the house, and you need to sleep. Grief is something you do between the moments of being busy and not allowing your pain to overtake you. Getting involved should be as crucial as any regular activity, but you don't have to make grieving into this big earth-shattering thing.

Being busy can create perspective in your life. Just don't use it as a way of hiding from yourself. While you should keep active, you should also remember and heal.

NO MORE "IF ONLYS"

Looking at all of the arrangements for my father's funeral, I was amazed by the vast flower arrangements you can order from flower boutiques or funeral homes. Surely, it would be better to give such massive floral bouquets to the living? But then I realized that these flowers were often symbols of regret. People buy lavish expressions of sorrow and the last gift given because they are stuck on "if only." They wish things were different, and they wish they had more time. The thing is, we usually don't have more time.

When my father passed, I desperately wanted more time to speak with him, tell him that I forgive him, and talk about fond memories. But, time had flown, and there was no getting it back. I was overwhelmed with thoughts of "if only I had spoken to him," "if only I had forgiven him when he asked for it last." "If only I hadn't been so darn stubborn and stopped making him suffer." And "if only I had known he would pass so quickly." I was stuck in time on October 17th, 2003, the day of his death. I never thought time would be up for daddy so soon at 62 years old! My biggest "if only" was not giving him the forgiveness he so desperately wanted from me. I had to let it go. ALS had killed my father, and my regrets were killing me. Not only had I not given my daddy the forgiveness he wanted, but I also didn't forgive myself. Putting my "if only" in the garbage where it belonged became the moment of acceptance for me.

I had to learn to let go of those "if only's" the regrets of not doing, and that meant becoming conscious of my thoughts and cutting them short when they turned down this dark path. Regrets and "if only" become like a vampire, sucking the energy and lifeforce out of you and leave you just a shell of your former self. Letting the regrets go will bring you back to life. If you're a stubborn person (like I am), get adamant about feeling better and live by not allowing the life-sucking "if only's" control every fiber of your being.

EMBRACE THE STAGES OF GRIEF

We have become quite familiar with the Kübler-Ross stages of grief model since it has been popularized in film and TV. While the actual model is based on interviews with the terminally ill, this theory still has excellent value. It states that we go through different stages of grief when we are facing loss (Holland, 2018). These stages include:

Denial

When you have suffered a severe loss, it feels like you have had the rug pulled out from under you. You are falling, and you can't believe it has happened to you. One minute you are fine and living your life, happily married, and the next, you may be divorced or a widow. When I lost my son, I went through such terrible denial. Even when I held his tiny body and gazed at him lying there so perfect in every possible way, I couldn't accept that he was not alive. He looked like he was peacefully sleeping.

Denial hit me big time. I went through various emotions: anger, fear, rage, regret, and ultimately, I experienced vast amounts of denial. For sure, the doctors were wrong? How could my perfect baby not be alive? I had done everything right during the pregnancy, so how could this have happened to me?

Your brain is trying to wrap itself around the idea of your loss. While your brain is a phenomenal organ, it doesn't always respond well to sudden changes, the loss being a prime example of that. So, you end up wanting to deny it happened. The shock eats at you, and you can't and won't accept that you have just had the most precious thing in your life taken from you.

So, how do you stop denying your loss? What can you do instead? For each of you, it will be something different. For me, denial only ended when I opened myself to feel my pain, acknowledge what had happened, and let the thought enter my mind that things had changed. I had blinked, and my life became a different version.

My father died in a mere two days, my son just short of seventeen weeks of pregnancy. Loss doesn't make an appointment with you. It doesn't schedule a time that suits you or a person you can "do without." It simply strikes. Accepting that it was inevitable and what time we have with the people who matter to us is the beginning of the grief process.

If you are in the denial stage, you may say things like:

> *No, he's not dead; he's just pranking me.*
> *My husband is just upset, and he won't go through with the divorce.*

*My friend is just angry, and we'll hang out again
once she's cooled down.*

These are all examples of denial articulated. Your brain isn't ready to change because we were comfortable, so it looks for reasons not to. By accepting instead of denying, you can change these statements to:

*He has died, and I know it will be painful to deal
with this.*
*My husband is not kidding, and we are really
getting a divorce.*
*My friend is upset, and it looks like we may not be
friends anymore.*

Acceptance isn't easy, and sometimes, when we can't, that's also okay. Even if you verbally admit to what has happened, it still allows your brain to internalize your loss. It would help if you started processing your grief. There isn't a prescribed period since it varies on our acceptance. Once you do, this often leads us to the next stage of grief.

Anger

Sometimes anger isn't anger. It may be sorrow disguising itself as anger or rage. You lash out at people who offer to help because you don't want to think about what happened, never mind having people around you see you suffering. Soon, your brain may try to limit the damage. Like you would lose the feeling in a limb that is injured so you can look for help, you may end up resenting the person you lost so you could "minimize" the damage of their passing from your life.

Sadly, anger also clouds your thinking (numbs you like that injured limb), and it stops you from being logical. Your husband's death is utterly sad. No, it's not the end of the world, although it feels that way. Eventually, you will be okay. People lose partners all the time, and then they move on and survive. You will too, once you start to process. Harsh as that may sound, and not to hurt your feelings, it is a reality to be conscious of your emotions.

Life goes on.

When you are so caught up in the anger stage, you may seek to chase people away from you, trying to create space for you and your grief to coexist together. You don't want anyone to tell you what to do or how to feel—you're hurting, and you won't have anyone tell you otherwise (right?). You may say things like:

> *I hate my father, and he was a horrible parent.*
> *My husband was a pig, and I don't need to be*
> *married to him.*

If God is so great, why did He let my baby die?

As you can see, anger and denial are often intertwined, and you may end up being both resentful and angry at the same time as you start processing your pain.

Instead of saying angry and hurtful things, you can try to bring some logic into your thinking, self-talk, and conversations:

> *My father and I had our difficulties, and his passing saddens me.*
> *My husband wasn't always supportive of me. And perhaps the divorce is a good thing.*
> *God is great, but I don't understand why my baby had to die?*

You can move through anger and begin to sprinkle in some acceptance and healing. Mind you, these are all just seeds at this point, and you will have two more difficult stages to go through before acceptance can flower. Be patient with yourself. I can't stress this enough. It takes time to cope, adjust, and move to the next stage of the grieving process.

Bargaining

After the initial denial and anger, you will experience a very human reaction: bargaining. That is your brain trying to solve the problem of your loss. By nature, your brain is an efficient organ, and it learns from mistakes. So, if you put your hand on a hot stove, your brain will ask why, and it will create a warning for future use: don't touch a hot stove. It burns. With the loss, your brain will seek to understand it. So, it begins reasoning with statements like:

> *If only I had been a better daughter, I would have ensured Dad went for regular health checks, and we would have found the disease earlier and treated it, thereby more prepared.*
> *Had my husband been more satisfied at home, he may not have strayed, and we wouldn't have ended up getting a divorce.*
> *If I had just stayed in bed all day, I might have given birth to a healthy baby.*

All of these statements are "if only's." They are only there to express what you wish had happened and how you think it could have changed the reality you now face. If only's don't work. They only torture you and fill you with the regret that you should've done something different and are self-blame. You can't control other people's actions. Sometimes we aren't meant to understand why something happens, and by endlessly trying to figure it out, we are just driving ourselves bananas. Instead of saying "if only," say:

> *The loss of my father saddens me deeply, and while I don't understand why this happened, I will focus on my good memories of him.*
>
> *My husband and I were happily married for a time until we weren't, and I believe our divorce may be better for both of us.*
>
> *I did my best for my unborn child, and I can only accept that they weren't meant to live.*

When you take away the "if only's," you are left with the reality of loss. At the same time, the loneliness, anxiety, and pain hits you even harder, often causing you to fall into, what I call, situational depression. When the situation changes into a more positive environment, the person is no longer depressed.

Depression

This can be one of the darkest stages of grief. You may feel like you wish you had traded places with the person you lost. You may want to join them in their passing. At times, you may feel like your life is over. It isn't, however, and you deserve life and happiness. I feel your pain because I've been where you are now, and it can be scary.

Depression is a terrible mental state to experience, and it can become long-term or even permanent if you don't take proactive steps to counter it. This period is when going to grief counseling and attending workshops on personal development are most important. You're at the lowest of lows, and you need to find new ways to build yourself up. You are most likely dealing with mental fog, fatigue, and confusion, which need attention. Don't just try to muscle through or bury it. Stop, feel, and heal. The death of someone or a breakup of a relationship needs to be addressed even though it may be difficult. You can't effectively heal if you don't.

I drew immense value from positive affirmations and mantras at this stage of my grief process, and I would say these whenever I had a chance in the day:

> *My daddy taught me many things that I am grateful for, and I honor his memory by living right and "staying on the straight and narrow path."*
> *During my time with my husband, I had days of happiness and days of sorrow. I choose to remember the days of joy and step forward into the light each day.*
> *For almost seventeen weeks, I loved and nurtured my son, and I embrace that a higher power now holds him.*

You can beat situational depression if you move out of that moment in time that you have tied yourself down to, but you need to fight and have a purpose. You need to take care of and tend to yourself like you would a friend who is going through a dark tribulation in their life. Be the friend you need to yourself. After some time of letting the feelings rise, subside like the ocean's tide in your mind, and inside of your heart, you will be ready for the last stage: acceptance.

Acceptance

People think acceptance means letting go of your loss and that you now suddenly forget about the person you lost. It doesn't. You can't undo the past, and you can't simply pretend that person never existed merely because thinking of them brings you pain. It wouldn't be fair to them, and it's not suitable for you either.

Acceptance means you reach an understanding of your grief. It's when you finally let that grief settle and become a less dominant part of your life. The pain is still there, but it's not sharp or prevalent; it's more like an occasional pang of grief. You find ways to move on and live life according to your potential, not your pain. Like the way, I still to this day honor my son and my daddy. They wouldn't want me to suffer or to be that way. They would like for me to live a happy life

I love this phrase from the Bible: "This too shall pass." It has brought me much comfort, and while I understand that not everyone is Christian or even religious, these four words are universal and describe the process of letting go so beautifully. It will pass. You're stronger than you give yourself credit.

That doesn't mean the pain will be gone. It doesn't mean you can magically unfeel the agony of loss. Instead, it simply means it will fade into the background, and you will live and perhaps even be happy once you move out of the moment of the loss.

The Kübler-Ross stages of grief have helped many people understand grief and the process of letting go. Yet, what is misunderstood frequently is the cyclical nature of these five stages. You may skip a stage, or you may have to repeat it depending on your healing process. It's never simple or easy, but at least, with this theory, you can have some assurance that you will be able to move on.

ACTION STEP 4: WHAT SHOULD YOU STOP DOING?

Think of your day. What did you do today that you have been doing a lot of lately (pretty much since you lost that person you love)? Your brain is trying to find and make coping mechanisms, but it's not always entirely logical about it, and you may be doing things that don't help. Are you using "if only's?" Have you buried yourself in work with no time to think and feel? Perhaps you've isolated yourself, as mentioned earlier, fearing that people will make you feel and think about your loss again?

Find the things you do that may be blocking the energy of your grief. Like a river, grief needs to flow through you. Only then can you begin to heal.

In your journal, write down how you have been blocking your grief. Ask yourself this question. Then write down why these things aren't helpful to your grieving and healing process. Instead of avoiding them, start releasing. Instead of hiding or burying them, start healing.

You are finally starting to look past the pain and into the heart of your grief. Inside you are the seeds of healing and growth. It's time to look there.

5

WHAT'S INSIDE?

I'm still coping with my trauma, but coping by trying to find different ways to heal it rather than hide it.

— CLEMANTINE WAMARIYA

When you have suffered a loss, it can create a trauma that isn't physically visible. You become frozen in the past moment, unable to be in the present time of now. You internalize with replaying the event in your mind, sometimes looping it over and over, becoming blind to everything else. You begin to carry the hurt with you as if it just happened as I did with my childhood trauma and my daddy's death. Looking inside can help you find the way forward, and it can help you find your feet when you have fallen back into grief. You can find new and alternative ways to cope with the pain of loss, but it is often overwhelming.

Trauma can be debilitating, with an array of symptoms of depression such as anxiety, appetite, and sleep pattern changes to panic attacks after "triggered." A song, car, or even a scent may bring those feelings to the surface as if they're brand new, flooding your body with cortisol stress hormones. There are ways of coping and getting past them that remove the emotional aspects of the event. It enables you to live in the present moment while not being emotionally tied to the past. In my situation, using every tool at my disposal, from journaling to techniques, assisted me in getting past the trauma and living in the moment of today. The past can only hurt you if you allow it.

HOW TO STOP BEING OVERWHELMED

After I had suffered several personal losses in my life before learning how to get past it, I began to notice that each loss was a bit like a pair of scissors that trimmed my fuse shorter and shorter. Pretty soon, I started snapping at people, really reacting instead of taking action. I didn't know how to step forward with calm and assurance. Instead, I felt utterly overwhelmed, and I couldn't find a way to break through and just breathe again.

Being overwhelmed is like having someone keep your head under the water, slowly drowning you no matter how hard you fight. It is a terrifying and painful experience, and finding a way to stop being overwhelmed can help you. It's how you stop snapping and become the reasonable and human person you are.

All of this snapping is due to you trying to hold on, hold back, and hold down by what you feel threatened. Sometimes, you need to lose control. You need to rage, rant, and cry. This can only happen when you stop feeling overwhelmed and start letting the force of your grief carry you. In the words of Blossomtips.com (n.d.), you have to "let it have its way" with you.

Like a fragile leaf that manages to survive the flood tide by simply floating, you need to let yourself get swept away for a time at least. This statement goes back to that "scheduled" grief. If you feel overwhelmed, then really let that feeling take you and run its course, and when it calms, you will be more resilient for having weathered the storm. Find a safe place like the shower, at church, the temple, or in the company of a good friend, and let yourself be overwhelmed. If you have nobody to be with you, then keep your journal with you and write while you let the storm sweep you. This is you allowing a natural process to happen, cleaning your mind's house and sweeping your heart clean.

Understand that while you feel overwhelmed and you may fear that your grief could drive you insane, it won't, and you will survive it. Grief is as natural as breathing. It's not something to avoid like a plague. Instead, you can look at it closer and figure out where your grief fits into your life. You may have moments of being triggered that happen quite unexpectedly where you see something that reminds you of your suffering. It can cause you to feel like you are drowning in grief again suddenly. That is also natural, but you can prepare for these by having a strategy for coping prepared.

How will you deal with:

- *The sight of a car that looks just like Dad's.*
- *A boy with blonde hair and green eyes that remind you of your child.*
- *The sight of a happy couple when you are just about to go through a messy divorce.*
- *Being unemployed while people around you are swiping and smiling as they spend money you don't have.*
- *Feeling lonely and seeing two friends hanging out and laughing happily.*

These are all triggers that can cause your sorrow to flow. They don't make appointments, and you can be blindsided suddenly at any time of the day. You need a way to deal with them without flying into a fit of tears and sobbing.

Maybe you can practice taking a deep breath while choosing to reflect on the comment, image, or other triggers that affect your grief at a time that suits you better? You could even create a habit of saving your feelings for the quiet times at night when you are busy writing or meditating to process a feeling you experienced during the day. Realize that you don't have to feel everything right when the feeling happens, but you do need to let it out at some point. This is healthy. And it is much easier when you do so daily at a time and place that is safe and encouraging for yourself instead of bottling it.

I would use a calming mantra to help me when I felt like I was drowning, like I was about to be overwhelmed: Right now, at this moment, I am okay. Tonight I can let the grief and negative energy go. That helped me focus during the day when I needed to be productive, and later when I had time to grieve without society watching, I could let it all out, rinsing my soul-wound with tears and a flood of energy.

By choosing to control when I felt, I could let go of what I felt, and it was empowering in itself. This was how I could stop being overwhelmed. Sometimes we take baby steps, and that is alright as well. A large part of this was also possible due to the reassurance that I had good people around me to help and support me.

ACCEPTING SUPPORT FROM OTHERS

You are not alone. I'll repeat it. You are not alone! There are people in your life who want to help. They want to be there for you, support you, and help you in any way they can. This is a cherished gift, and you should accept that gift with grace and gratitude. Don't slap away a helping hand as they try to show sympathy and being empathetic.

If people want to share what they have to help you up, then accept their efforts. That is not, by any means, says that you are weak. Since the dawn of time, people have been helping each other. We can still see this in all "primitive" cultures where traditions of several hundred years in the making surround their grieving rituals. From taking food to someone who has suffered a loss to simply comforting them, we can all relate to another human being somehow. This is precisely the support we need. It reminds us that we are not alone, and we can turn to people around us for comfort and support. You don't need to have multitudes of people for help. It could be one person or several since the number doesn't matter. What matters is that you have someone to give your moral support and assist you emotionally through this trying time.

Sadly, in modern society, we often fear accepting help as gossiping and that public opinions may result, and so, we try to struggle through the quicksand of grief alone. When you are sinking, you need to let others help you.

At the worst of times, I was fortunate enough to have a loving family who was there to help me up. I had been blessed with wonderful friends whose sisterhood meant the world to me during my grief stages, and without these, I would not be where I am today.

You have support; know them, find them, and use them. Let your support network in. Over time, you will begin to heal, and you can then pay your support forward. When you have been through grief and grieving as I have, you can then help others when their time to walk with sorrow comes.

THE GIFT OF TIME

They say time is a healer. That is true, but only when you put in the work. Wallowing in self-absorbed misery and pain isn't going to help you heal—no matter how much time you give it.

Use the gift of time to help you heal. All wounds will heal over time if you apply the right kind of dressing to the injury. Likewise, you will heal over time if you create grieving rituals and let your emotions become fully experienced. You are applying medicine to your wounds, and this period will be effective.

Over the days, weeks, and months, your hurts won't seem nearly as bad as you have developed perspective. This is what heals you. Over time, you start to think differently about your loss if you have done the work. You can redirect your focus from the loss to what you need and who you still have in your life.

The gift of time is your friend that brings wisdom and makes you stronger, equipping you with tools to deal with other life situations. At some point, someone may come along amid a crisis that is very similar to what you've survived. You can then be their beacon of hope and comfort and give them the empathy they need to provide them with the fire to move ahead.

YOUR POSITIVE FEELINGS HAVE POWER

Being positive can help you cope. This may sound like a no-brainer, but people often forget they have the power to pursue and embrace positivity. Being positive is not something you magically are; it's an action you can choose to do.

Your thoughts have the power to choose positivity, which will, in turn, lead to a positive feeling. Consider these examples:

Instead of thinking ...	Try thinking ...
<ul><li>I'm so lonely after my boyfriend left, how will I be able to face this day?</li><li>I'm so sad after losing that person, and I don't know how I will cope.</li><li>There's no way I can carry on now that I am single again.</li></ul>	<ul><li>Today is a beautiful day, and I have the power to choose with whom to share it.</li><li>Losing that person is sad, but I am resilient, and I can carry on.</li><li>I embrace every challenge as an opportunity. I will thrive.</li></ul>

ENGAGING IN SELF-CARE

Taking care of yourself is even more critical when you are grieving. There is nothing noble about "suffering publicly." People seem to believe that they are the noble grieving widow or widower by denying themselves basic self-care. News flash: You deserve better, and I'm sure they wouldn't want you living for their death. Within a breakup, caring for yourself and your appearance would be the best route to take. Your former partner may want to see you distraught, so be happy, and find other things that bring you joy.

Begin caring for yourself. That means you need to take care of your basic needs. Have you been:

- Sleeping enough?
- Are you eating healthy?
- Drinking enough water?
- Getting some exercise?
- Connecting with friends?
- Reading good books?
- Taking time out to simply sit and breathe?
- Kind to yourself?
- Creating opportunities to laugh?
- Letting yourself cry through healthy means, like watching a good movie?
- Taking yourself away for a change of scenery?
- Dressing comfortably but not hanging out in your PJs all day?
- Practicing gratitude?
- Saying no to things that don't serve a purpose in your life?

Self-care is important. It's what makes life a little easier, and it is about being kind to yourself. You deserve it.

YOUR ROUTINES CAN SAVE YOU

When we've suffered a loss, we expect the world to stop and stand still because ours has. It doesn't, though. This frequently is what seems the hardest to deal with when you are grieving. I remember wondering at one point after my father's death how the world could just keep going on when he was no longer there. It just didn't make sense to me. And so, for the longest time, twelve years to be exact, I struggled to move on. It seemed like there was no point to the day, yet I had to cook, clean, look after kids, and be a functioning member of society, despite my world no longer spinning. I was stuck at the moment and living for his death, not celebrating his life.

That is where I discovered temporary autopilot, and it helped me get through days when I couldn't think anymore. When grief had so clouded my judgment that I couldn't see or think or feel, I could rely on routines to keep me going. While I didn't want to get out of bed because so depressed, I did. I didn't want to eat, but I did. I didn't want to take the kids to school, but I did. At times things may not seem to matter, but they do. Like the cliché, "fake it 'til you make it."

Regular routines helped me structure my day and just get through them. I'm not saying the pain went away. No, that was there alright, and I had a terrible agony of spirit inside me after the losses I had suffered, but I could function. I could get up, make sure the kids were ready for school, and pack lunches if need be before dropping them off and carrying on with my day.

For a while, I disappeared into the details of my life, but I didn't grieve. I tried ignoring my grief by burying it. Of course, this didn't work because burying it, as I discovered later, was the worse thing to do. Instead, I felt more and more depressed. But then, one morning, I went through a box of some old photos and found one of my daddy, and the tears began to flow. So, I started a morning ritual where I would spend five minutes with my grief. If I wanted to cry, I did. When I felt sad, I might write a few lines, and when I remembered a fond memory, I allowed myself to laugh. When I recalled a memory with daddy playing the piano singing, and I joined in to harmonize as he had taught me as a little girl, I smiled, then I would think of other happy memories with him. I realized that the feeling of guilt lessened.

I made my grief a part of my routine, and slowly, I began to heal because I dealt with it. The guilt became less, and I was no longer running from my pain or regretted not telling him that I forgave him for everything when he was alive. It became a part of me, and suddenly, it wasn't so raw and terrifying. I began replacing the sad memory with a joyful one.

ACTION STEP 5: HOW ARE YOU COPING?

What have you done to include your grief in your life? We are so quick to try and push the grief aside like it's interfering with our lives. But really, grief is a part of it. It's the opposite side of joy, and you shouldn't deny it. So, in your journal or downloading the free Wellness Workbook :

1. Write down your triggers that make your grief raw and also ways to deal with these.
2. Who is your support network? Write down the names of the people you can depend on. Who can you turn to for a glass of wine and a giggle to lift your mood? Do you have someone you can talk to seriously about your feelings? Perhaps there's a person whom you can turn to when you need to get away or get out of the grief space. Identify and value them.
3. Reflect on how time has begun to change your perspective and how healing has begun.
4. Become mindful of your thoughts. Are they positive or negative? Is there a recurring thought

that dominates your mind? Write it down, evaluate it, and find a mantra to counter any negative ones.

5. Where are you on your self-care scale? Do you look after yourself? While it's good to spend some time each day reflecting on the person you lost, you should also spend some time each day thinking about yourself.

6. What routines can you create to help you focus and function? How have you integrated your grief into your routines?

7. Have you forgiven yourself? Forgiveness is such a powerful tool that we can wield. Forgive yourself for all of the "if only's" and even forgive the one that left the relationship for whatever reason.

If someone chose to walk away from you, forgive them. It may be difficult at first, and you don't have to say the words to them. You can write in your journal or write them a note or text. After my divorce, when I told my ex that I forgave him for how he treated me during our marriage, the hurt left, and I was happier. Only then did I realize the magnitude of burdens that I had carried up to that point. I realized just how much energy it took to have negative thoughts and feelings against him. When someone has done something to hurt you, and you carry that hurt or negativeness with you, they don't feel the pain; you do.

It's effortless to simply wish the loss never happened, that the pain you feel never existed. But that would be an even more significant loss. By embracing your loss, you can change your life to help the healing and grieving process and ultimately make you a better person.

6

FOCUS ONLY ON CHANGE

The first step toward change is awareness. The second step is acceptance.

— NATHANIEL BRANDEN

When you are ready to start your healing process, you may want to rush headlong into the experience. Take your time because you deserve it.

To heal means you will have to change. This change will drive you towards the healing process; it creates the inward peace we all seek. Like that cut I had on my finger, grief isn't something that can heal overnight. It needs space, time, and forgiveness. You need to practice self-forgiveness and let go of being a victim. The power to heal is in your hands.

CREATE SPACE

Space is not only physical; it's mental and emotional too. It would be best if you gave yourself the time and opportunity to feel bad. That may make no sense, but it is also perfect sense. When you allow yourself the time and space to feel bad, your emotions can realign themselves. According to a study by Hershfield et al. (2013), when you let bad feelings have their time and space to manifest, you limit the long-term damage these emotions can cause if you try to suppress them. Take the bright with the sad, and you will be able to live a wholesome and balanced life.

Over time, as you create the space for letting bad emotions air out, you will find your overall health improving, and you will develop something many people never have—wisdom. You can even go so far as to have a unique space allocated for your sad feelings and self-reflection. Perhaps you have a chair set aside by a window with a view, or you keep your journal nearby so you can write about painful feelings when they happen. Give yourself the space and time for all of your emotions to be acknowledged. That is how you get to really know yourself and discover your strengths.

BEGIN FEELING

You may have tried to hide away your pain. Certainly, nobody wants to feel anguish and sorrow. These emotions hurt, so we hide them away, trying to continue living as if we never felt those emotions. But we do feel them. Sometimes they feel so amplified that it feels like we're teetering on the edge of a cliff.

Only once you start letting those feelings out can you begin to have a whole and complete emotional footprint. This will require you to adopt a view of welcoming all your emotions, whether they are happy or sad. You can comfortably face each emotion since you know it's not your only emotion. While you may be unhappy at this moment, you know you can and will feel better soon.

If you notice you are feeling sad or upset, you can try the following steps to help release that energy (instead of avoiding or suppressing it):

Let It Flow

Your instinct may be to jump up and try to distract yourself, but if you feel upset or sad or any other negative emotion, stop and let yourself feel it. Take a few minutes to sit and simply feel what you are feeling. If you are sad and want to cry, then do so. You discovered earlier in this book the benefit and reason for tears. Let that emotion run its course. As the saying goes, 'just go with the flow."

Release the Energy

Then, take a few calm, cleansing breaths and let yourself settle in this moment of time. When you are ready, find a transition activity that releases negative energy. It could be to go for a run, a walk, or take a hot bubble bath. You could even turn up the volume on your car stereo and sing at the top of your lungs to something such as Linkin Park's Hybrid Theory album, as I did. Whatever you choose to do, let the draining energy of those negative emotions go.

Do a Mindshift

Now that you are starting to step out of the negative emotion, it is essential to do a mental shift. Go out and collect leaves, bake something for your family, or take up a new hobby. Find something positive produces recharging energy to help you change your negative emotions into positive ones. This statement goes back to what I said in an earlier chapter from Oprah's tv show about replacing negative emotions with one more positive.

NOBODY HAS THE RIGHT TO TELL YOU HOW TO FEEL

We are often looking for more "knowledgeable" people to tell us what to do in life. Making decisions is a scary process, and when it comes to dealing with grief, we tend to do the same thing. You may find yourself tempted to listen to people tell you what to do, even when what they say doesn't resonate with you. When dealing with my loss, I received some pretty unhelpful advice that had no benefit for me while it may have helped someone else. Perhaps you received some "wise nuggets" like these:

- When I lost my brother, I simply packed his stuff and my feelings into boxes. By boxing up your life, you can get over it.
- I heard that grief only really lasts a year, but you've been angry and upset for five years, so what's wrong with you?
- To deal with grief, you need to be so busy that you can't waste time on it.

Needless to say, these statements were made by people who meant well, but the brutality of the words and the bluntness of the ideas were (and are) entirely off target. While I can't imagine anyone benefiting from such thoughts, the worst part is believing you can tell someone what to do.

Nobody has the power to tell you what to believe, what to think, or how to feel. You decide what to choose or how to react. Your feelings are within your hands.

SELF-FORGIVENESS

Like in Chapter 4, when you are faced with a devastating loss, you may be tempted to engage in "if only" thinking patterns. These don't help, and in the end, you may start blaming yourself or resenting the person that has left your life. After all, it is human to look for someone to blame. Inevitably, you will blame yourself.

To change, start practicing self-forgiveness. Would you hold someone else responsible for a loss that wasn't their fault? No? Then why do so to yourself? Why hold yourself accountable for what you could not control?

A good friend shared a little gem of wisdom with me shortly before I finally came to terms with my dad's death. She said: "What would you tell me if I were in this kind of situation? Would you tell me that I was to blame, or would you tell me to forgive myself?"

That was a real lightbulb moment for me. How would I advise a friend this but not myself? Should you not be your own best friend? And, at that moment, I decided that I would let myself off the hook. I would finally let myself practice self-forgiveness.

You can do this too. Simply think of yourself as a close friend whom you care greatly about and let go of the blame.

POWERFUL STEPS FORWARD

When you finally reach the point of no longer holding yourself responsible for what you couldn't do anything about, you will be ready to start moving forward. It can be challenging since you have lost all forward momentum in your life. Being in limbo emotionally may mean that you have reached inertia mentally too.

To move forward, you need to develop some skills that will help you calm the floods of pain and emotional turmoil so you can hoist your sails and catch the winds of life. Here are a few ways that you can gather speed in life and travel onward on your journey:

Affirmations

When you have suffered such terrible loss that your brain seems to be stuck in the same gear each day, you will notice your thoughts are often repetitive and negative. You can see this with the kind of self-talk you are engaging. Do you think to yourself that you are strong and resilient and you will make it through this challenging time, or do you think that it's all gone to the dogs and that you will be unhappy and lonely forever?

Should you notice repetitive negative thinking, you need not be harsh or unforgiving to yourself. Instead, simply let yourself find joy and compassion by swapping out the negative with positive affirmations. Here are some examples:

Negative Self-Talk	Positive Affirmations
• I'm not good-looking enough, which is why they left me.	• I am beautiful inside and out, and I live my life happily.
• My father's passing has left me so sad and lonely.	• I had the blessing of spending time with the person I loved, and I am grateful for that.
• I feel abandoned by my friends and family due to my pain.	• Noticing how my family supports me, I can stand tall.

Positive affirmations will help you change your mindset and reach inner peace and change instead of drowning in pain and sorrow. You can make personalized affirmations;

remember they are always written and spoken in the present tense and first-person. Affirmations are never negative; always try to be positive and let your emotions carry you forward. By controlling the inner self-talk positively, the negative comments said to yourself will change. A core principle in therapies is changing the self-talk from unhelpful and damaging statements to more productive and positive.

- Today, I release the pain and exhaustion from my body and mind.
- I have given myself the time, space, and permission to grieve, and I am ready to move forward and be happy.
- Grief is only a tiny part of my life, and I am whole when I let myself live fully.
- I choose to hold onto love and memories as I let go of pain and negative self-talk.
- Today, I take stock of my feelings and acknowledge what I have been through while rewarding myself by taking a break.

Yoga

Moving your body is a great way to get yourself more physically in tune and boost your positivity. Movement helps your body produce endorphins, and these are what helps you feel good. Any activity will do, as long as you enjoy it, and it cares for your body. While I chose to do yoga and dance, you might decide on light Callanetics or walking or running. You'll know you have chosen the proper movement when you feel good after a session, and you start wanting to do it more often.

Yoga and slow, meditative movements like tai chi help you enter a calming mental state, a double bonus. While moving your body, you can also move traumatic memories from your mind, letting them go and entering a healing state. Additionally, yoga combines well with meditation practices like Vipassana, which can help you trigger a release of your body and mind.

Journaling

Throughout this book, I have been urging you to write, pour the pain you feel onto paper, and use this to help you release your emotions to begin and guide your healing. In the beginning, it can be intimidating to start writing. There is something about a blank page that can be quite off-putting to a first-time journaler. If this is you, you might consider getting a journal with writing prompts or using a journaling app to help you break the ice. Online subscription services will send you daily journaling prompts to help you open up and write. You can also start by asking, "What do I feel today?" "What positive statement can I tell myself?" Or, "To regain focus today, I will….?"

I also started what I call my thought jar. It's a screw-top glass jar that I keep on my desk. When I think through the day that worries me or triggers a memory I am not ready to think about, I quickly scribble it down on a slip of paper and add it to the jar. When I have my quiet time writing and reflecting at the end of the day, I use these slips as prompts to help me recall what concerned me today. I can then calmly use my journal to give the memories and grieving space to be resolved. If it was just a negative feeling or thought at the time, I drop it into the trash if I no longer feel that negative statement. Sometimes it may just be ranting, but the symbolism of taking it out of my head and putting it onto paper is enough to be free of it

Using my journal or thought-jar, I can make my grieving part of my daily routine, and I can feel like I am productive and constructive with my feelings. This gives my loss meaning and helps me be a stronger and more resilient person.

Art

When you are trying to find your way forward, you need to express yourself. Sometimes, we simply don't have the words for this. The pain runs so deep that we can't articulate it, and we just can't release how we feel. That is where art is a powerful ally. If you can't speak, then paint. When you can't write, then draw. And if you can't discuss, then sculpt.

Whether you are painting faces on pebbles or using oil on canvas, any art is a form of powerful expression, and you should let yourself use it to get the hurt out so you can look at it, make peace with it, and move forward. Many artists do this same thing to cope with what they feel, seen in their artwork.

Talk About It

Moving forward means finding ways to let go of the painful past. Yet, it's not something you can just dump and run away. You may find great benefit in talking to someone. Whether this person is a therapist or a caring friend you feel comfortable talking to, it doesn't matter, as long as you find someone who will give you time to talk, without them feeling the need to try and solve your problems.

During these conversations, it is a good idea to talk about your plans on how to accomplish moving forward and not only focus on what happened. Sometimes, all you need to move forward is to hear yourself say that you are doing it. Hearing your plans articulated can be a tremendous motivational force, so use it.

Another and alternative way to heal is to share and help others with their loss. I experienced this first hand after leaving the hospital after my child's stillbirth:

I had experienced some difficulty getting pregnant again after the birth of my first child, and after a four-year struggle, I was thrilled that I was finally pregnant. While it was not an ideal pregnancy as I had placenta previa, where the egg implants near or onto the cervix, my baby was thriving according to the ultrasounds and developing. We found out it was a boy, and we decided to name him Brandon Christopher. I started bleeding, although the doctors didn't know why. Still, he continued growing, and the doctors put me on strict bed rest except for daily ultrasounds to keep an eye on my son. The doctor had me skip the Thursday in-office ultrasound the following week and have the more detailed ultrasound that Friday. Every day, the ultrasounds had shown Brandon moving about and healthy despite my bleeding. I realized before the appointment that Brandon wasn't kicking like he usually did in the mornings. As I watched my son on the big screen at the scan, my heart broke. The doctor confirmed that my baby had died. At just short of seventeen weeks, my baby was dead. Something had happened, and he had started bleeding. It was a painful and unfair mystery. Doctors explained my body would naturally proceed with a miscarriage over the weekend. It was the longest weekend ever! I couldn't bring myself to attend my husband's buddies get together, knowing I would be asked questions from the other wives about the pregnancy or want to feel him kick. My body echoed what I wanted and was not letting go of my precious boy. I was scheduled to induce labor early on Tuesday. It was such a long day of Pitocin dilating me. At 10:05 pm, I gave birth to my stillborn son. I insisted on holding him, and as I cradled his small and perfect body in my hands, looking him over, I felt so utterly abandoned at that moment. My husband was unable to deal with the death, refusing to even look at our son as he sobbed uncontrollably. I felt that he almost blamed me for my body's failure to carry a healthy child and give birth to him as God had intended. Why my son?!

Having those days over the weekend to come to terms helped my grieving process before Brandon's birth. After seeing my nurse-midwife, who talked to me extensively, she asked that since I was mentally doing better than expected, if I could speak with a couple of ladies who had also just lost their babies. In all, eight other women had miscarried, some at eight to nine weeks and others at seventeen weeks as I had. In sitting with those

> *bereaved women, who also felt like their worlds*
> *had ended, I began to realize the value in sharing*
> *the pain. In that precious tear-stained moment of*
> *sharing, there was a sense of no longer being alone.*
> *Suddenly, I had sisters I had never met or known*
> *before, and we felt a shared understanding of*
> *belonging.*

Sharing with others, taking a moment out of your own grief to help someone else breathe in theirs, is often a powerful way to find a purpose. You are helping someone else live and find hope, although you feel like you have lost yours. Whatever your loss, you are not alone in it. Others have also lost, and their pain is as real as yours. By sharing that pain, you may find the grip of desperation loosen just a little so you can take someone else's hand in friendship as I had at that women's clinic.

RELEASING VICTIMHOOD AND EMBRACING VICTORY

Moving forward entails letting go, but it also means knowing what not to hold. When you choose to hold on to your pain and the loss, you are placing yourself in the role of victim. With being a victim comes a whole bag of tricks that may be strangely appealing to you. For starters, when you are a victim, you will receive sympathy, attention, and expressions of comfort. Within doing this, it can make you feel special, and it can be pretty addictive.

This may sound harsh, but if you are honest with yourself, part of not moving on is because you don't want to stop receiving all of the attention. That doesn't mean you wished the loss to happen. It simply means you don't want others to move on with their lives while you are stuck in yours. Being a victim is easy. Becoming a victor is so much harder, but it is the way to rise above the flood tide of pain and loss to become a ship in the storm to others.

ACTION STEP 6: DO YOU HAVE INNER PEACE?

To heal from loss, you need inner peace. It can be hard to know whether you have it or need to work at achieving it. Indeed, this chapter can serve as a kind of checklist to help you evaluate your inner peace.

In your journal, reflect on the following questions:

1. Have you embraced change in your life?
2. Did you make your space a reflection of your life now, free from loss and the past as you head into the future?

3. Are you letting your feelings reveal themselves?

4. Do you practice daily self-forgiveness and attention rituals?

5. Have you used affirmations, meditations, journaling, yoga, and movement therapy to let you open up and talk about your loss?

6. Have you left victimhood in pursuit of victory?

7. In your recovery process, you may be letting go an inch or finger at a time, and while you have made good progress in finding peace and letting go of pain, you still have a distance on this recovery road to cover. There's more than just letting go.

7

MORE THAN LETTING GO OF RELATIONSHIPS

Remember, we see the world not as it is but as we are. Most of us see through the eyes of our fears and our limiting beliefs, and our false assumptions.

— ROBIN S. SHARMA

Healing after a broken relationship or a loved one's death is about more than letting go. It's about really acknowledging your feelings. You need to let your emotions become free of the pain as you need to heal from your pain and loss. That means you need to learn about what you are feeling and how to process your emotions. If you don't acknowledge your feelings and keep shutting them away, you will soon find your feelings dwelling in an empty space in your heart. Letting your feelings out is like increasing the blood supply to your soul so you can heal. Like any wound, you need to clean it, care for it, nurture it, and let it sometimes air out. That is the healing process part that is going on.

EMBRACE YOUR FEELINGS

When did you last value your feelings? Have you talked profoundly and intimately with your feelings, letting them manifest in fullness in your mind and heart? Most likely, you are not letting your emotions out. That can lead to the area around your soul wound becoming necrotic and rotting away. If your living experience is not adequately nourished by soul-affirming tasks like writing, making art, creating poetry, or moving your body kindly, then you will be like a septic wound that is starved for air and care.

Embrace your feelings. Value them, even the ones that aren't all that pretty. When I lost my husband in our divorce, I didn't feel all that pretty on the inside. I felt ugly. It didn't matter that it was my choice to leave an abusive relationship; I still felt unwanted. My feelings were a mix of resentment and pain. And since he was the father of my three daughters, I felt like I had to hide how I felt about this loss. Needless to say, when you hide your emotions, they become rotten. My resentment became something gruesome to see.

It frightened me, and I wanted to try to pretend that I didn't feel what I felt. Then, one day, as I was writing away in my journal, I had a moment of deep and lasting peace where I took a long hard look at my resentment and anger. I allowed myself to look at what I had been feeling and, most importantly, why I was feeling it. Without judgment, I managed to see the anger and pain that had created these feelings of resentment, which were from years of "it" balled into one. I asked myself whether the reason for this feeling still existed and how I could let it go. I was no longer in maltreatment, called any names, or told that I was things that weren't true. I had to check in with myself and ask, why continue to feel a way that didn't represent the current situation? I'm no longer there and have the ability to make a conscious shift for a more positive outlook. Although I missed it at times, our marriage died, it was over, and I had to move past.

Each time I felt that growling anger inside me before, I treated it like a sad puppy, and I would mentally stroke its head and then tell the feeling that I no longer needed it. It didn't seem logical to continue crawling down that dark path when it didn't serve me to feel that way any longer.

IT'S NOT ABOUT WHO IS RIGHT

This section can and may be tricky. We don't like to be wrong and admit that the left is right, flowing both ways. Losing someone can make you feel like you have to compete with the person you love or loved. You were once equaled and could share. You may now be opponents and want to win over the other. With exes or family members who leave, you may find the arguments particularly painful and exhausting.

You may be wanting to show who is right (believing it's you), so you can somehow win and be okay. Here's the truth I realized: There is no winning. Trying to prove you were right will not make you feel better. Making the other person be this horrible, unworthy loff of a person will not help either. Loss is loss, and you can't undo yours by trying to win over the person or trying to get the last words in. It doesn't serve any purpose other than ego, even if you want to throw more word daggers because you're hurting and angry. It's hard to be the "better person" and play nice when you just want to tear them to pieces. It's a waste of energy and won't help your healing process at all, even if there's the possibility of feeling a little bit better afterward. In the long run, there aren't any benefits to doing this. All it does is create an opposing force within you that you continue to feel shadowing and overtaking any joy around you.

DEVELOPING INSIGHTS: YOU CAN'T CHANGE OTHERS

When I was in the midst of my divorce, I wished so sincerely that I could somehow change my husband and make him see what I had been through with my past of not feeling secure. I tried explaining to him so many times about my feelings and how the experiences I had been through had shaped me, including his demonization of me, but he didn't understand. I tried explaining that his quick temper was to blame for his screaming instead of talking to me, and his actions were the culprit for losing my trust during our marriage, but it didn't matter.

This left me feeling alone and very isolated. I wanted to convince my husband to see things my way, but I couldn't. He didn't understand, and he probably never will. So, it was up to me to accept that I couldn't change him into being what I needed and wanted, so our marriage was over.

When you are dealing with loss, you may want to change the other person. We can only influence people through our example, but we can never change them. We all are unique, and when someone doesn't support or thrive with yours, it makes a difficult decision.

Holding onto someone we aren't supposed to be with and who may not be part of our journey ahead can be an act of desperation not to be alone or try to avoid more loss. You can't change people, and not all loss is terrible.

A relationship ending due to infidelity may make you feel insecure and blame yourself for it. Infidelity is one of the most prominent causes of breakups, with the communication breakdown a substantial factor. If you are letting go in this instance, you may feel betrayed, unloved, undesirable, or that it was somehow something you did or didn't do that was the cause. Acknowledging that you can't control other people's actions is the key phrase to your healing. Another person's actions are there's alone. You may begin to question yourself, asking where did I go wrong? Could I have prevented him from being unfaithful? What did I do to deserve this? Here's the naked truth; people do what they sometimes do without provocation. There may be nothing that you could have done differently to change the outcome.

The decision to no longer be in a relationship with that person due to broken trust starts with your acceptance. Deciding to leave the person you love is extremely difficult, and you need to do what's suitable for you within your situation, with or without children. The end of a relationship goes through all of the same phases as death. Coming to terms that you can't change them or the dynamics will be a key to your healing.

Loving someone isn't enough to avoid loss. I loved my son, but I couldn't change his fate. You may love your spouse as I did my husband; your love can't change that loss. Accepting and embracing that you can't change people to avoid loss is a moment of liberation. Suddenly, you can see and love the people you fear losing all the more, and you can choose to let go of the people who no longer resonate with your life and your soul.

ANALYZE YOUR FEELINGS FOR WHAT THEY ARE

Pain is an influential teacher. Sometimes we don't let go because pain makes us fearful. Even though what lies ahead and the future may be positive and better, we may hang back since we fear loss. Letting go of pain and loss may cause you to feel abandoned. This can be worse than the actual pain.

It would help if you analyzed what you feel and what they reveal about you. When you fear being abandoned by people in your life who were with you during the initial stages of loss, you start to cling to the past, as looking to the future may be more intimidating.

I think of the first loss I suffered and how convoluted my feelings and experience of the loss. I had intertwined my identity so profoundly with the other person I lost that I couldn't move forward. I began carrying the life of the person who died. That can be a massive load to shoulder.

So, I had to distinguish what emotions were mine and which belonged to the person I loved and lost. Hence, I began to:

Disentangle My Emotions

I like to use visualizations to help me with complex tasks, and seeing myself as different from the person I lost is one of the hardest things I ever had to do. I had to keep reminding myself that it wasn't some form of judgment or punishment that I was using against that person. Instead, it was simply about getting some perspective and seeing my life and what was theirs.

One visualization I used was to picture a clear mountain pool with a smooth and glassy surface. Every so often, a drop would fall from above to splash into the pool, sending out ripples that faded outwards until the bank was still once more.

I was the pool, and the drop was the other person's impact. It was traumatic when there was an initial energy exchange, and the ripples would circle through my life. But, when I let myself become still, I could regain my inner peace and be only myself.

Next, I visualized a small wooden bucket that I placed suspended above the pool. With this intervention, I could catch the drops, and I didn't have to suffer the disturbances of energy entering my life. I could avoid becoming involved in the other person's dramas and overflow damaging to my calm.

This technique is beneficial for people who have to say goodbye to someone they love but are no longer suitable for their lives. With my divorce, I heavily relied on this technique to bring me calm and peace. I also realized that when I remembered painful events or even happy ones that could upset my tranquility, I could use the bucket to catch them to later look at them without them rippling through my life.

You get to decide what things go into constructing your bucket. Is it your faith, self-belief, meditation, journaling, habits, or rituals that let you catch the drama without having to look at it right now? Whether or not you let that drop reach the surface of your calm is up to you.

Evaluate and Improve

Loving someone isn't enough to make them stay in your life. I loved my husband, but in the end, our marriage was on the rocks and ended in divorce. It can be unclear, draining, and mentally taxing when you have given it your all, and things still didn't work out. You let that person whom you still love go can be a devastating loss.

It makes no sense, and you may wonder what the point of it all is to be in a relationship at all. That is where you need to start evaluating and look for ways to improve future relationships. Every single event in your life is there to help you learn, grow, and heal. It isn't about pointing fingers and saying the other person is to blame or about trying to convince yourself you didn't love them in the first place. There's no sense in lying to yourself to change how your heart feels. Instead, it's about learning more about who you are.

Again, don't look to find flaws in yourself. Nobody is to blame for a relationship ending, and while the loss is challenging, you shouldn't try to shoulder the blame or assign it to someone else either. For a time, there were two different personalities in the mix. Attempt to look objectively at the situation and see what you can learn from it. You could question yourself:

- What did you do that worked, and what about the things that didn't?
- Were there patterns of behavior you could learn from and guard against in the future?

- Did you miss signs, or did you simply not put in enough work?
- Were you honest with them about your feelings and concerns, or did you say nothing, hoping the situation would work itself out?

Accountability is about doing what is needed, being answerable for what you do, and showing up to be present in your relationships. You author your relationship book, and it's up to you to turn pages or look back and learn for future chapters.

Avoid Assumptions

The loss of a relationship is tough to handle as you may find yourself constantly wondering what went wrong. You may torture yourself by thinking about what may have been happening in the other person's head. You may wonder what they are thinking to leave you and turn from being someone you love into someone you loathe.

Here's the real kicker: You don't know what they are thinking.

Don't assume you know what is going on in their mind. While I had moments of believing my husband was the worst possible person after everything I had been through, I had no idea what was going on in his head. I may have assumed that he was thinking unkindly of me or that he had no respect and no love for me, but I didn't know what was on his mind at the time.

Likewise, if you are suffering the loss of a relationship, don't assume you know what is driving it. People don't always want a divorce or break up because they think less of the other person. Their inadequacies feature strongly in their decision-making, and their decision to leave may have more to do with them and less to do with you. It may hurt to think that someone would leave you, making you feel that you are the cause. The brutal reality was that it was all about them and their perceptions and not ones about you.

The same goes for the death of someone. Wondering what they thought of you, or did they know how you felt about them, can leave you feeling stuck and weepy. Having lingering questions or answers and dwelling on them will stunt your healing. Case in point, like not telling my daddy that I forgave him when he had asked for it countless times. I assumed that as he lay dying and knowing it, he probably thought that I didn't love him at all. Taking on assumptions of what the other person may have been thinking will only add to your frustration and more friction.

After losing their child, a husband who leaves his wife may do so because he feels like a failure and can't stand to see her suffer. Perhaps he left since he wants her to be happier and, with their constant fighting, believes he is to blame for their marital conflicts. You don't know, and asking someone what's going on may not produce helpful answers either. Sometimes, we don't even know what we are thinking of ourselves. Our emotions are tumultuous, and we drown in the confusion of our feelings. So, we may let go simply to avoid dragging the person we love down with us.

Wish Them Well

Here's the hard part. How often do we hear about someone who has lost a partner, and when they speak of that person, they seem to be vomiting up bile? They are so bitter that it is painful to listen to them talk about the person they once loved. Avoid poisoning yourself with bitterness.

Let go. Allow the person to move away. Disentangle your emotions from theirs, and when you have let the person move out of your life and from your feelings, wish them well. Yes, wish them well.

It's not helpful or healing to curse and swear and tell them to f*** off. This is a person who was part of your life, and whether all the time with them was good or bad, you have been changed by them. So, let them go, let the anger and negative emotions with them, and allow them to continue with their life journey and prosper.

This is equally important if you are divorcing and have children with them. It is difficult to bite your tongue and not say what's really on your mind with children in earshot. I about bit my tongue off from the temptation to tell him just what I thought, and it can be very stressful for everyone. Trash-talking the other parent either with the kids overhearing or directly to them could backfire. This one may prove to be particularly difficult to accomplish, having raw feelings so near the surface. Your children may end up protecting the other parent who is talked about negatively.

Kids need to feel that they can love you both without having to choose sides. I understand you may not want them to love the other parent or even to like them, I felt that too, but it wouldn't be fair to force the kids to choose. When my daughters experienced this, along with mudslingings from their father, it made them angry at him for doing so. It didn't matter if there was a sliver of truth in anything he said; he attacked my integrity and character, they felt the need to protect me, so it backfired on him. I leaned on my faith and writing in my journal to pull the negativity out of my head, so it didn't fall out of my mouth.

With that said, kids are resilient and may appear to handle everything fine when they are dying inside. If you have divorced parents, then you know how they feel. The two people they love most in the world will no longer be together, and the children may become insecure or begin to have behavioral issues. Becoming absorbed in our drama, we may forget that the children are hurting or feel worse at times. There are knowledgeable family counselors that can assist in the transition to prevent or resolve problems that they may be feeling. Small children as young as two or three years old who don't have the tools to articulate how they feel will show signs during their play and, a trained therapist will be able to assist them.

Find some way to release the negative emotions you may harbor through meditation or mindfulness (faith and alternative forms). Let go of negativity so you can release the person who is leaving your life

Don't Do It Alone

Loss is draining and energy-sapping. You may feel like you can't set one foot before the other. And depression is always a real threat when all the positive energy and good in your life seems to walk out the door with the one you loved.

This is when you need support. Get a support team together to help you manage the letting go and recovery process. When I say team, I do mean team. You can use your journal to write down who in your life can support you with what. That may seem cold and calculating, but it's simply using logic to help you when your emotions feel fried. The panic that sets in when you deal with loss can overwhelm your thinking, and you may end up with deeper emotional and psychological damage if you let it go on like that. Understanding which friends are there to cheer you up, which are there for weeping on their shoulders, and which are there to help you clear some brain fog and point you in a healing and helpful direction.

Just because the end of the relationship is your loss doesn't mean you have to do it alone. Others have walked this path before you, and if you let them, they can show you a few landmarks along the way.

If you are not as blessed to have many people in your life who can help you, or perhaps you don't feel comfortable confiding in those people, you can use therapists and online support groups like E-Therapy Cafe and Grief Healing. Wherever you look, find someone who can support you without ulterior motives, biases, and hidden agendas.

Redirect Your Focus Inward

Can you control your loss? What is in your power to control? Can you direct the actions of others or determine what outside people should do? No, the only person in your ability to influence is yourself, as said earlier. Any other attempt to make others do what you want is an example of manipulation. You won't have any real focus when you keep looking outward at others.

Keep your focus on your own life, the power you have to help change things, and your ability to accept what you can't change. That is how you limit the energy you lose by worrying about other people. Instead, invest your energy and efforts into what you can control and let the rest go.

Get Real

You may feel completely lost, so when you find someone else to step into your life, you may feel overjoyed, like your life has just begun again. Sadly, this can go two ways:

One: you are lucky, and the relationship deepens, fulfilling all your wishes with hard work and effort. Or, two: the relationship tanks because you are still stuck in the past. You are absorbed in disillusioned fantasies that don't lead to genuine relationships. Doing this requires self-care, and you need to meet your actual needs. You would also work on dropping any unrealistic expectations that may tarnish real and tangible happiness.

"You can't open the window until you close the door." Moving into another relationship quickly before you've settled your emotions from the last one may have a different outcome than you expected. Be realistic and genuine about your loss and not draw into how a future relationship will somehow be easy and perfect. You will only set yourself for failure. Many get drawn into the first person that gives them attention and skips part or all of the healing process. If you have insecurities, they will follow you unless you address them honestly.

Give yourself the much-needed time to heal, regain your balance of emotions and self-love so that you can face the subsequent relationship while standing on your two feet. Once you no longer dwell on your former person or relationship, you will be able to devote your attention to someone else, in all fairness.

Practice Kindness With Yourself

You have just lost someone with whom you probably thought you would spend the rest of your life. It is a terrible blow, and unlike other setbacks in life, this is a big one. This loss may make you question everything you believe about yourself. There is a reason that therapists say divorce is the same as death. Something has died: your "us" with someone you loved.

While you may want to power forward and be strong, you need to practice self-love towards yourself first. If you need time to rest, take it. Maybe you need space to grieve, create it. And if you want to talk, find someone who will be kind to you. When you are kind to yourself, you restock the well inside you from which you supply buckets of kindness to others. Kindness is like charity—it starts at home (with you), and you can send it out by doing good to others.

ACTION STEP 7: DO YOUR FEELINGS MATTER?

I hated how my feelings felt like a sin when I was grieving the loss of my relationship. I had somehow gotten it into my head that what I felt wasn't valid, that what I was experiencing wasn't as bad as I "imagined," and that I had to "grow up and deal with it." That denied my feelings. I had been cruel to my own heart and mind. Have you been in this boat? Did you also self-efface your emotional state and mental condition because you didn't believe your feelings mattered?

Stop doing it now. Your feelings matter. Nobody can tell you what to feel or how long you are allowed to feel it. There is no time limit on grieving, and one form of grief isn't "worse" than the other. I have experienced many forms of suffering, from losing a child, a parent to losing my marriage and my fiance', and they all hurt. Each is different and unique in its scope and magnitude. Nobody, including you, can tell you which is worse. It is simply one thing. It's a loss, painful, and life-altering. Whether or not you heal from it and make the experience a life-affirming journey is up to you.

To do this, you need to open up to your feelings. You should welcome them with open arms, let them explore and grow, and help them heal you. Yes, even the negative emotions can help you heal, but only if you let these out and give them the recognition and time they deserve.

Write in your journal about your feelings. Articulate, draw, paint them, or sing about them, but find a way to acknowledge your feelings and let them become released from the painful tightness in your life. It's time to start relaxing inside, letting yourself off the hook and healing the last of your scars.

8

THE PAST IS PAST

There is no revenge so complete as forgiveness.

— JOSH BILLINGS

After this journey, you are ready to let go finally. It is time to release the feelings and beliefs that have held you, prisoner, to your grief. Forgiveness is the last step on the road to healing and dealing. It's time to forgive yourself and the person you lost.

The best way to step forward using constructive energy is to learn from both the pain and the past. In learning, we can discover forgiveness and finally let our loss scab heal. Your orientation will change from despair to a growth-directed mindset. A real recovery is now possible.

FORGIVE YOURSELF AND FORGIVE THEM

"I should have" and "They should have" are typical statements of deep regret that are being articulated. We won't let go, clinging to the pain and not wanting to let go. But when you hang on, you stop the flow of energy in life, and you end up resentful and poisoned. The only cure for this is forgiveness.

Forgiveness. Such a simple word, but so hard to practice.

To let forgiveness work in your life, you need to start practicing presence and mindfulness. When you are present in this moment, this now, you can't think of the past where sorrow is. You also can't then live in the future where worry starts. Instead, you live here, right now, between breaths. That is where you learn only to feel this moment and take things one step at a time.

With present moment thinking and awareness, you will be unable to look at the vast issues you have become wrapped up inside. Instead, you will look inward at this heartbeat, this breath, this touch, and this space. You are here, you are okay, the pain is bearable, and your life is continuing. You can forgive anything outside of this moment as you are letting go. To help you along, I have a few favorite mantras to share:

- I can choose who I am at this moment, and I am proud.
- My past can be remembered in peaceful reflection, but I don't have to carry it with me.
- My life serves a greater purpose, and I learn from my mistakes.
- All that I need I have within me, and I am sufficient at this moment.
- I let light and happiness fill me each day so that I may shine it out to others.
- Right now, at this moment, I release what has been my pain point.
- From this experience, I have learned what I could, and I can now let it go to welcome new experiences into my life.
- My existence is one of light and abundance for myself and others.
- In letting go, I am made free from the past and all pain.
- I forgive those who have caused me pain, and I move beyond the loss by forgiving myself.
- I am stronger than I give myself credit.

Forgiveness starts with you by learning, letting go, and moving positively to the future.

STOP DAYDREAMING

One of the worst ways to trip up your progress forward is to let yourself engage in ruminations. Perhaps you find yourself recalling events or memories you shared with the person you have lost. That can be pretty energy-draining, and you will have to find a way to stop. Rumination may turn to daydream, and soon, you will end up wishing the person was still in your life. Yet, when you have lost someone, the chances of you getting them back and having a meaningful relationship with them may just be fantasy and wishful thinking.

In an abusive relationship, losing the person who was your abuser may seem ideal, but there was a time when they were kind to you. There will have been moments when you loved them. Wishing to have that again can be the road to hell as it may trigger you into running back to someone you really should lose. This is why women tend to leave their abusive partners many times before they actually go for good. The abuser apologizes, stating it will never happen again, drawing you back into their web of deceit. With this kind of thinking, you will be causing yourself needless harm. Nip it in the bud by stopping daydreaming and nostalgic recollections of "better times" as these are gone. All that lies before you now is the road ahead.

Let go, forgive the person and yourself, and move forward.

STOP BACKWARD THINKING

You have the potential for a beautiful life ahead of you. When you stop looking in the rearview mirror at the past, you can't see your future in front of you. Future thinking is what promotes growth. I'm not talking about fantasies of how wonderful and prosperous you will be once you win the Lottery here. No. This is the ability to visualize yourself in your future being happy by using what you have now. This is part of your goal setting. You should be able to visualize every step to getting you to this goal in your future. It helps bring clarity and focus into a life that may feel very chaotic at the moment after a significant loss. Write them down as much as you can. Write every detail that will pave the road to this happier self.

So, here's my future vision I created to help me let go and move forward into a healthy life that would make me happy:

> *I started by seeing myself happy and in a home where there was peace each day. In my vision, I participated in activities that made me feel good*

*about myself. Ones allowed me to bond with my
daughters and support their dreams with my own,
but not at the cost of my own.*

*My vision included details that unfolded as I
quietly sat and simply waited for my life to open
and heal. I saw my daughters as grown and confi-
dent women, and I saw grandchildren who played
on my knee as I happily bounced them. A deep
quiet started in my mind, and I could see myself
taking authority in my life.*

*By reaching out to other women who have suffered
loss, I see myself as able to help others and heal my
scars more and more each day. Positive energy
flows through me, and I am relieved from the
sorrow that had been weighing me down.*

*In my mind's eye, I can see my future. This is a
glorious destination where I am heading. When I
find a still and wonderfully peaceful moment in
my future vision, I pause and look around, taking
in all the joy I see in my dream. Now, I look backward, seeing the steps that will lead me to this
great victory. I take a small step back to the
beginning.*

*From experiencing momentary joy, I step back to
moments of sadness and pain and stepping back
further, and I see myself writing and managing*

the painful past. More steps backward reveal how I will communicate with the person I lost and manage the range of messy emotions I feel. I see myself learning new things, trying out different experiences to help my spirit remain positive. It's not always easy, but it is worthwhile to work. Finally, just a few steps above where I am at the moment, I see how I will begin forgiving the person I lost and myself too. I see how I will think of them less and less, and while I remain grateful for the past experiences with them, I let go of any longing to have things "the way they were," for this is not possible. I am heading into a new future now.

At this point, I usually open my eyes and feel a profoundly supportive presence all around me, and I believe my faith is restored and rewarded. Now, I know the path ahead, and I am familiar with the steps to walk. It's mapped out for my feet, and all I need is to walk along, for I will reach my future destination.

Your future vision may look different from mine. Whatever you see, be sure to focus not just on what your future will look like, but how you want it, and see how to get there. This is constructive forward-thinking, and it is way more helpful than negative backward thinking.

BE THANKFUL

I love the catchphrase that seems to be doing the rounds of having "an attitude of gratitude." How incredibly true this is. Being a spiritual person and someone whose faith has sustained her through the worst times, I do believe in "counting your blessings," and this is not simply another phrase to tape on your fridge or load as your status on Facebook.

Begin to practice gratitude every day. It's incredible how it can help you remain positive when things aren't going well. Studies have proven that being grateful and expressing it every day can help improve your mental health (Brown and Wong, 2017).

To practice gratitude, you can also use your journal. You can list three things in the morning that you are grateful for today and why. Then, before bedtime, you can again list another three things you were thankful for during the day and why. You can also write a gratitude letter in which you thank those who helped you become the person you are today. Try to be aware of the things that make you grateful to have. Being thankful for parents because they had you is sort of meaningless for future growth. But being grateful to your mom for being your pillar of strength while growing up is helpful and gives you a role model. You can also express gratitude for intricate things, but that shaped you and helped you become stronger. Even death can carry a certain amount of appreciation if you look at it from the proper perspective.

While I would give my stillborn son anything to survive, I am grateful for the time I had him when he was alive and the spiritual guidance and inner healing I received and achieved following his death. I am thankful to become a guiding presence to other women who suffered such devastating loss amid my own anguish. That experience had brought me so much closer to my beliefs and saw my faith renewed. It lit the way of what I believe is my purpose on this earth. It is why I sought more education to assist others in their life issues and complications. How could I not be grateful for it?

Gratitude is like a healing balm, and once you apply it to your life and experiences, it changes the way you look at everything. Then, everything about you can change for the better. While there is a lot of deep content in this chapter, and it's a lot to take in and apply to your life, practicing gratitude every step of the journey each day of your life can help you overcome loss and help direct you towards healing.

START MEDITATING

Meditations are about finding inner stillness, which is a good thing for anyone believing in a higher power as this means you are better able to hear your maker. So, I used meditation interchangeably with the concept of prayer, but the silent kind where you wait and listen for answers.

So, becoming still is a significant step forward in letting go of the past. When you are quiet, you can hear your thoughts, and you can ease them, releasing those that affect you negatively most.

I'd love to share a simple meditation I do daily to help me let go of the last shreds of worry and pain of the day.

Sitting in quiet allows your body to become comfortable and at ease. Let your mind slowly settle and become like a tall tree that is gently swaying in the breeze. It is perfectly balanced, and whether the wind is gentle or fierce, the tree of your mind is never uprooted or perturbed.
As you inhale, you notice how the tree gently sways to the left, and as you exhale, you see the tree swing to the right. It and now you are so entirely balanced at this moment.
While you are watching the mighty limbs gently

weave in the wind, you notice there are a few
branches that have broken from the lower reaches
of the tree. Some branches are dried and will fall
soon. These are the events from your past that
have no purpose to your tree anymore.

Intentionally, you start to remove each of the
dying branches, noting that each has a name. You
discover worry, jealousy, and resentment first.
Gently pulling, they tumble to the ground. Other
more negative emotions and memories follow as
dried branches that you have shed.

Your tree is not lessened by these branches falling
away. If anything, it is inspired to grow taller and
broader still. These branches no longer serve any
purpose, and it is good that you remove them from
the tree.

As night falls, you drag the branches closer and set
a bonfire. Lighting the dry wood, you sit in the
glow of the bright fire as your past and painful
memories burn away in warm flames. The light of
the fire reflects off your tree, lighting it up against
the dark sky. You are also mesmerized by the
showers of sparks that fly off into the air as the
fire crackles. These sparks are the little moments
when you will recall your past moments in the
future. Note how briefly they flare before being

extinguished again. You need only wait and watch them. There is no need to interfere, and you are utterly at peace.

Looking at the ash from the fire, you know tomorrow you will add this to the tree base to help fertilize the soil and help your tree grow stronger still. You learn from the ashes of your past and grow more and more into the great and dignified living being you are.

A FEW LAST POINTERS

As I wind down this chapter, I want to share the last few pointers to help you on your path to healing. Firstly, I want to look at the myths that do more harm than good. These are the things society wants to comfort you with, but if you listen to this kind of reasoning, you will not release your burdens nor heal your hurts.

Pain Goes Away When You Don't Look at It

What a terrible myth! Pain can't go away when you ignore it. Only by acknowledging it can pain be healed and released. Buried things still run in the subconscious mind running in the background and remain fresh as the day it happened. It also can bring forth symptoms such as anxiety that you may not realize why.

Look at your pain. See it. Allow it to stand in the light where you gently embrace it and then let it slip back into your past where it belongs.

Being Strong Is How You Cope

Sometimes we aren't meant to be strong. To build ourselves up again, we may need to break down to become a small heap of disjointed parts. Being assertive can stop you from grieving, and you may end up with an even bigger wound inside that may never heal.

Loss is debilitating, so when you want to, feel broken it doesn't mean you are broken for good. You still have the power to pick yourself up. But trying to hold yourself upon a foundation that is now missing will not help you achieve release.

Those Who Don't Cry Are Not Coping or Dealing With Loss

Not all everyone can cry. Sometimes you cry on the inside, or you are too busy resolving your emotions to cry. You may also only need to cry once or a few times instead of being a wailing mess all the time. Nobody can tell you that you aren't dealing with your loss. Only you can know if you are busy processing, resolving, and internalizing your loss.

Forget What Happened So You Can Move On

Letting go and forgetting is not the same. Forgetting means you don't learn from something, and you avoid thinking about it. But really, that something is always at the back of your mind, often torturing you. Moving on is an adverse action in which you run from your past. Instead, try moving forward and letting go of the pain that you place behind you.

LOSS AND GRIEF CHECK-IN

Now that you know your options to approach grief and grieving, you can better process your loss, deal with it, and begin to heal. However, it is worth doing a check-in to make sure you are on track. Like a doctor checking symptoms in their patient, you need to check in with yourself and gauge whether you are really healing or if there are still unresolved issues to deal with it.

Emotional Check

- Have you moved from the shock and disbelief of the loss to a place of acceptance, and can you now realistically look at and talk about the loss?
- Can you express your sorrow in meaningful ways, like crying or investing your grief into some creative outlet?

- Do you feel guilty for a part of the loss? Have you forgiven yourself and let yourself off the hook for what you may initially have believed to be partly or all of your fault?
- Did you let go of your anger, letting it drain from you to leave you free to allow healing to begin?
- Are you facing your fears that the loss may have triggered, or do you turn away?

Physical Check

- Are you still feeling tired or stressed?
- Do you experience bouts of insomnia and nausea with frequent illnesses striking you?
- Have you gained or suddenly lost weight?
- Do you feel listless or disinterested in routine activities like eating or personal hygiene?

FINAL CONCEPTS

As a last parting word, I would like to also speak on two very complex issues that we often ignore when grieving. It is essential to be aware of these and know a little about them to ensure your healing is a natural and flowing process.

What Is Complicated Grief?

When your grief doesn't seem to improve, and it's been several months since the initial loss, you may need to consider that you may be suffering from what is known as complicated grief. During normal grieving, you will experience good days and bad days, and while you still feel sad, your suffering will lessen slightly with each passing week.

Sometimes, we don't seem to get better, though. Our grief becomes a festering sore that doesn't heal no matter how much time and energy we put into self-care therapy. This is a sign of complicated grief.

When I first heard this word, my initial reaction was to say, "isn't all grief complicated?" Yet, this specific form of grief is intense grief that dominates every aspect of your life long after your loss happened. You may become unable to function, work, to look after your family or yourself, and you may feel completely overwhelmed and stuck.

Watch out for the following symptoms manifesting as they may indicate complicated grief, which can result in post-traumatic stress disorder taking over your life:

- You are thinking about your loved one every moment of the day to the point that these thoughts and daydreams about them interfere with everyday activities.
- You see your loved one everywhere, which may become hallucinations if your mental state is further disturbed.
- Being in such denial about your loved one's death, you start forming outrageous conspiracies to explain that they are still alive somewhere.
- Intense avoidance of anything associated with your loved one.

- Suffering extreme bouts of rage and anger at the loss.
- Struggling to find any meaning in life.

Suppose you are suffering from several of these symptoms. In that case, you may need professional help, and you may also need chemical intervention to help you cope with the floodtide of emotions you may be suffering. Ask for help when you need it because there is no shame in it. The body is not designed or built to be on high alert all of the time. It is your life we're talking about and your mental health. There is nothing noble about suffering alone and in silence for the rest of your life. Remember that life is for living and not for grieving.

Are You Grieving or Suffering From Depression?

Grief can be rather depressing. You may wake up some mornings and wish you didn't have to get up and face your pain again. Still, most of us slowly find our feet and carry on, learning to cope with grieving. Yet, some of us are so overwhelmed that we slip into total depression, which is a psychological condition that requires careful management as it can affect brain chemistry. Prolonged stress hormone release can accentuate an already severe issue.

When you are manifesting the symptoms of depression, look out for the following:

- A deep sense of guilt, like death, was your fault.
- Thinking about death, dying, and suicide often.
- Have a complete loss of energy throughout the day.
- Lack of motivation to do any activities.
- You're feeling inadequate and hopeless.
- You're hearing or seeing things in hallucinations.
- You're not bathing or eating as usual.
- You have been experiencing these feelings continuously for two weeks or more.

Depression and grief aren't the same, although symptoms may be the same. When you are suffering from depression, you require medical intervention. Be conscious that grief may change into depression if you leave it untended and unresolved.

ACTION STEP 8: ARE YOU PAST YOUR PAST?

So, here's the final kicker. It's time to see if you are ready to let go.

In your journal, write a letter to the person you lost. Reflect on your lives together, their method of passing from your life (either through choice or by death). And finally, thank them and wish them well as explain why you are letting them and grief go from your life and that you forgive them and yourself. If there was something, they wanted or needed to hear from you that you refused to say, write that down. If you regretted doing or not doing something, and it is why you are having difficulties getting past their death, write that down. See this as final parting words.

When you have written the letter, place it somewhere safe or close to your journal and don't read it for a few days. Then, when you feel ready, sit somewhere quiet and read your letter aloud. It is essential to hear the words in your voice. This is you giving yourself permission to let go and move forward. It may make you emotional listening to your words, and that's okay.

Evaluate how you feel with each sentence being read and let yourself become immersed in the words. Do you feel a weight lifted from you or feel a deep shudder inside like someone is ripping out your heart? If it's the first, then congratulations, you are progressing well on the path of healing and self-recovery. If it's the second option, then you are not ready to let go. You're not on a time limit. Perhaps you may need to rework some of the tasks in this book, waiting a few weeks before rereading this book and learning the values and insights anew. You can master your pain, as I did. It is possible to find peace and a way to let go finally. Don't give up! Focus on healing every aspect.

Be kind to and forgive yourself as you gently guide yourself on this journey. It isn't a sprint, and it isn't easy, so don't be too harsh on yourself if you don't quite feel ready to let go of your loss. This person impacted your life, and perhaps you just need more time. You may have only loosened your grip on your grief this round, but you can work on it more. Nobody can tell you how long the journey will be, but you can walk it, and you will begin to let go, heal, and become whole again.

CONCLUSION

We must let go of the life we have planned so as to accept the one that is waiting for us.

— JOSEPH CAMPBELL

One of the hardest things to do is accept that what we had planned on isn't in our future at all. When you lose someone, the world you had imagined for yourself suddenly is crushed. Whether that person has suddenly died or has decided to continue their journey on their own (or with someone else), your life and your potential aren't over.

You can journey onward into a bright future. However, this journey is much easier, quicker, and more enjoyable if you're not weighed down by the pain, uncertainty, and anguish of your loss. Your life experienced a bad chapter, and you are not a bad book.

I hope this book has guided you on the first steps to finding inner peace, letting go of what pains you, and discovering your path ahead. Your life isn't over; it's just beginning.

Grief is a process, whether it's death, divorce, or a breakup, and now that you know the steps in that process, you can begin to change and let go of that which you can't change. It's time to accept the life that is waiting for you. It is a beautiful life filled with potential and promise. All you need to do to grasp it is free up your hands by letting go of the old life you are burdened with and taking hold of your new destiny. It is a destiny of positive energy and compassion with yourself and with others.

Letting go of the person you love may be the best step you will take, but it will also be the hardest one ever. Yet, you have it in you to deal, heal and forgive after loss so that you can finally regain control. You were a complete person from the start, and they only added to that. Relight your candle and shine brightly into the world with eyes forward and both feet under you. You are a beautiful soul that deserves happiness, joy, and love.

"You are stronger than you give yourself credit." It may be challenging to start, but you need to focus on your well-being and normalcy.

I hope that you enjoyed this book. This book has been a year in the making and very close to my heart. While writing the last chapter of this book, I suddenly lost my aunt, my mother's baby sister, to cancer just a day after being diagnosed. As you can imagine, it was quite a shock to my whole family. The statement that I heard the most is that they wished that they'd had more time. It should make us more aware that we never know when the time is up and value those we love cherishing every moment with them. I used the same tools that I have described within this book to help deal with the loss.

I do hope that you can heal. It won't be overnight, and it will be a painful process, but it is worth it in the end.

As an author with a small publishing company, reviews are my livelihood. If you enjoyed this book, I'd love it if you left some feedback. I love hearing from my readers, and I read every single review. Your review also helps others to find this book and a way to heal from their pain. Thank you so much for reading!

Other books by Julian Demarco that you may like: Listed by Amazon as #1 New Release in Self Help categories: Transpersonal Psychology, Inner Child, Mental Illness and Hypnotherapy.

Understanding Childhood Trauma & How To Let Go

11 Effective Tools You Need To Heal (By a Fellow Survivor)

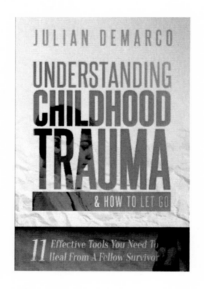

An excerpt from an editorial review from "booklife reviews" on Amazon:

"Demarco's openness will resonate with trauma victims, particularly in the recounting of past sexual abuse and the dangerous relationships that stemmed from early

traumatic experiences. She offers a sage advice, "just because I had left the abusive environment didn't necessarily mean the record of abuse had been cleared from my mind." Though the bulk of the guide addresses specific therapies and exercises for recovery, Demarco makes it digestible even for entry-level readers by offering clear examples and breaking more complex topics into easy-to-follow steps.

Clinical professionals will appreciate the boots-on-the-ground analysis of treatment options, while readers will welcome the empowering messages, like the recommendations to "let go of the belief that perfection equals happiness" and to open up to significant others about their roles in the healing process. The overarching insight that trauma recovery must be individualized, with no set timetable for healing, pairs nicely with Demarco's goal to help readers "reclaim control" over their thoughts. The end result is as informative as well as inspiring."

REFERENCES

Billings, J. (n.d.). *Josh Billings quotes.* Brainy Quote. https://www.brainyquote.com/quotes/josh_billings_121409

Branden, N. (n.d.). *Nathaniel Branden quotes.* Brainy Quote. https://www.brainyquote.com/quotes/nathaniel_branden_163773

Brown, J. & Wong, J. (2017). *How gratitude changes you and your brain.* Greater Good Magazine. https://greatergood.berkeley.edu/article/item/how_gratitude_changes_you_and_your_brain

Campbell, J. (n.d.). *Joseph Campbell quotes.* Brainy Quote. https://www.brainyquote.com/quotes/joseph_campbell_386014

Cherry, K. (2021). *The benefits of being open-minded.* VeryWellMind. https://www.verywellmind.com/be-more-open-minded-4690673

Deschene, L. (n.d.). *40 ways to let go and feel less pain.* Tiny Buddha. https://tinybuddha.com/blog/40-ways-to-let-go-and-feel-less-pain/

Dyer, W. (n.d.). *Wayne Dyer quotes.* Brainy Quote. https://www.brainyquote.com/quotes/wayne_dyer_384143

Finley, G. (n.d.). *Guy Finley quotes.* Brainy Quote. https://www.brainyquote.com/quotes/guy_finley_513816

Hershfield, H. E., Scheibe, S., Sims, T. L., & Carstensen, L. L. (2013). When feeling bad can be good: mixed emotions benefit physical health across adulthood. *Social psychological and personality science,* 4(1), 54–61. https://doi.org/10.1177/1948550612444616

Hesse, H. (n.d.). *Hermann Hesse quotes.* Brainy Quote. https://www.brainyquote.com/quotes/hermann_hesse_384604

Holland, K. (2018). *What you should know about the stages of grief.* Healthline. https://www.healthline.com/health/stages-of-grief

Irwin, T. (n.d.). *Terri Irwin quotes.* Brainy Quote. https://www.brainyquote.com/quotes/terri_irwin_902544

Laurie. (n.d.). *What to do when grief overwhelms you.* Blossomtips. https://blossomtips.com/coping-with-setbacks-feeling-overwhelmed-grieving-process/

Mann, N. (2011). *The health benefits of crying.* Netdoctor. https://www.netdoctor.co.uk/healthy-living/wellbeing/a10637/the-health-benefits-of-crying/#:~:text=Stress%20release&text=Higher%20levels%20of%20adrenocorti-cotrophic%20

(ACTH,health%20problems%20associated%20with%20stress.

Sharma, R. S. (n.d.). *Robin S. Sharma quotes.* Brainy Quote. https://www.brainyquote.com/quotes/robin_s_sharma_857685

Walters, B. (n.d.). *Barbara Walters quotes.* Brainy Quote. https://www.brainyquote.com/quotes/barbara_walters_119104

Wamariya, C. (n.d.). *Clemantine Wamariya quotes.* Brainy Quote. http

s://www.brainyquote.com/quotes/clemantine_wa-mariya_917522

Made in United States
North Haven, CT
31 October 2022

26135713R00114